the HEALTH CARE TEAM Book

the HEALTH CARE TEAM Book

TIM PORTER-O'GRADY,
PhD, EdD, FAAN

Tim Porter-O'Grady Associates, Inc.
Atlanta, Georgia

CATHLEEN KRUEGER WILSON,
RN, PhD

President and Senior Partner
Specialty Applications
Phoenix, Arizona

Mosby

St. Louis Baltimore Boston Carlsbad
Chicago Minneapolis New York Philadelphia Portland
London Milan Sydney Tokyo Toronto

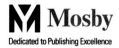

Mosby
Dedicated to Publishing Excellence

A Times Mirror Company

PUBLISHER
Nancy L. Coon

EDITORS
Lisa Potts & Yvonne Alexopoulos

ASSOCIATE DEVELOPMENTAL EDITORS
Aimee E. Loewe &
Kimberly A. Netterville

PROJECT MANAGER
Dana Peick

PROJECT SPECIALIST
Catherine Albright

MANUFACTURING SUPERVISOR
Don Carlisle

BOOK DESIGNER
Amy Buxton

ILLUSTRATOR
Chris Sharp

Copyright 1998 by Mosby, Inc.

ISBN: 1-55664-504-X

Printed in the United States of America

Composition by Mosby Electronic Production
Printing/binding by R.R. Donnelley

Mosby, Inc.
11830 Westline Industrial Drive
St. Louis, Missouri 63146

To Mark, whose inspiration and dedication to growth and to building partnership serves as a beacon to all whose lives he touches

To Mardie and Tom, whose lives are a reminder to live fully in each day and to make the choices that advance the quality of our own lives

To Andrea, sister and best friend, who works with love, respect, and caring in all that she does; she leads by her example

TIM PORTER-O'GRADY
CATHLEEN KRUEGER WILSON

Preface

Anyone in health care who is unaware of the major transformation currently underway is either dead or has been living in a cave for the past two decades. There is no person in health services who has not had a personal experience or felt the impact of the redesign, downsizing, reconfiguring, and integrating of health services.

Many books have been written over the past decade on change in health care and how to confront it, challenge it, mold it, or manage it. There are more than sufficient resources available today to assist in dealing with the vagaries associated with such a major change. In addition there is much written on what the changes imply for the future of health services, including several written by the authors of this text.

As health services move toward a much more integrated and continuum-based approach to service delivery, a new mindset around the nature of work and the processes associated with it becomes critical to sustainability in health care. With the recognition that teams are the basic unit of work comes the demand to retool the workplace to build on team processes rather than continue to focus on individual roles and behaviors.

There are many implications for the organization in the move to team constructs:

- Focus on the individual now becomes the obligation of team members rather than of the organization's management.
- Performance evaluation now is a team process looking horizontally at each team member and his or her contribution to the work of the team.
- Focus on work now shifts to viewing outcomes rather than process alone with the understanding that there must be a tightness-of-fit between the two to create truly value-driven results.
- Resource considerations now must be a part of everyday clinical decision making.
- More often decisions must be made in the same place where they will be implemented and by the same people who will implement them.
- Relationship becomes more important than control in ensuring effectiveness in a horizontally linked service structure.
- Systems are membership communities rather than employers enclaves demanding inclusion and empowerment as a part of the operating milieu.

The workplace is not the same place the majority of us entered into in the initial days of our work experience. The conditions and circumstances that define work and prescribe it are much different from what they used to be. We can no longer assume that the "old" rules for work are viable and that we can depend on them to define the parameters or content of work. The "teaming takeover" is a response to a different context and a new set of needs in place and necessary to support the requirements of work.

Teams require a different format and framework to ensure their viability. Much of the effort in the next two decades will be centered on creating the conditions, processes, and structures that support the use of teams. New behaviors will be required to ensure that the dynamics of the team are promulgated and outcomes sustained. Structure and process will have to converge to provide the supporting context for the continuous and consistent achievement of outcomes. This interface between supporting structure, effective process, and defined outcomes becomes the defining interface necessary to support the work of teams.

The work of the time is to prepare people to live within the context of teams. Changing focus and relationship is clearly a significant task on the part of every worker who finds himself or herself in the throes of adapting and working within a team format. Becoming a team is just the first step in a series of experiences that will transition the style, process, and intersection of work into a different formula for success. The diversity and interaction that is necessary to thrive in this set of circumstances is challenging to say the least. The work of the time is to prepare the worker to not only live within the context of team relationships but to be able to become a fully invested and participating member of the team and to build the relationships necessary to thrive there.

This TEAMbook is designed to provide some of the initial tools necessary for both teams and members to thrive in the context of teams. The focus here is not only on skills and adaptation to team living and working but also on the environment, context, and structure necessary to sustain teamwork. Many books address behavior and skills for and of teams; however, few of them spend any time on the structure and organizational framework necessary to sustain teams. The authors believe that this interface creates a more comprehensive support for helping organizations and people adapt to working within a team framework.

Creating teams is much easier than sustaining them. Many organizations for a team approach and spend many hours and resources on making them work. This TEAMbook is designed to simplify the process of development by focusing on the key variables essential to the team-building and team-maintaining process. The tools included in this book are designed to assist team leadership in the development of essential elements and characteristics necessary for an effective and continuously functioning team. These tools include the following:

Focus boxes to target specific, supplemental information and considerations that are essential to management.

Notes in the margins about the health care system, teams, definitions, and so on that supplement information found in the text.

Team Tips to provide helpful hints for team members.

Words of Wisdom to give sound advice to team members.

Tool Chests that include team-building tools to provide specific, practical help in forming and operating within a health care system.

The goal of this TEAMbook is to provide the key elements and processes on which teams can build real effectiveness and support their ability to continue to thrive.

No resource is sufficient alone to inform the reader with all that is necessary to sound action. This TEAMbook serves as one tool that, when combined with other resources, provides a database the reader can use to expand understanding and application of concepts and processes that ensure good team development. The authors believe that the key elements essential to successful team design and process are enumerated for the leader in a way that can be effectively applied in any setting.

Health care institutions are unique. Team development within the health service framework is not the same as that which unfolds in the business service arena. The unique service needs imbedded in creating a healing relationship and environment require a specific application of team process and format. The caring environment so necessary to generate the healing elements between provider and patient and within the patient requires a specific sensitivity and application of the team dynamic within the care continuum. The key theme of this TEAMbook centers on the healing relationship and the healthy interactions necessary between team members essential to meaningful health service across the service continuum.

The need for constructing the continuum of care, creating the essential linkages, and building the relationships and behaviors necessary to ensure good outcomes flows through each page and chapter of this book.

This is an exciting time in health care. The landscape for building real health-based approaches to service provision is shifting daily. The foundations for building partnership and accountability in teams are consistent, however, and simply require that the principles be consistently applied to the formation and functioning of teams. This TEAMbook provides those foundations and can serve as a valuable tool in the successful implementation and operation of teams within any health care setting. The authors hope that it will be a valuable handbook in the leader's armamentarium of developmental resources for creating and functioning in teams.

Tim Porter-O'Grady
Cathleen Krueger Wilson

Contents

1 Transitions and Transformations: Making Sense of Change in Health Care

Change is not a season; it is a way of life.

Anonymous

BEGIN AT THE BEGINNING

This is not a book about change. Instead, it is a text that helps us deal with change. Almost any book or article written on health care topics today deals with understanding or explaining the changes that are happening all around us. This book does not intend to do that. Instead, we assume that you understand that change is occurring and are in some way involved in creating response to it. What is needed, therefore, is some help with how to do that.

BUILDING A FOUNDATION

This chapter provides a backdrop for translating some of the changes into a language and framework that the reader can begin to apply. We take a look at what is unfolding and begin to get a picture of the circumstances of the change and a stronger idea of the appropriate response to it.

The problem with the current change cycle is twofold. First, so much change is occurring that it is difficult to sort through it; second, this change often is filled with such complexity that becomes difficult to find the key elements that serve as the driving forces for the change.

Change is a constant; it never stops, nor does it ever go away. To manage change you have to first embrace it.

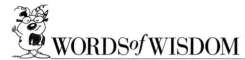

WORDS *of* WISDOM

We are experiencing a world change. This means that everything in our world is undergoing significant shifts. The challenge for each of us is to search for the meaning that lies at the heart of the changes and ask ourselves how it impacts us and what will be our response.

~

Real Change
• Is sustainable
• Builds on the past
• Affects behavior
• Addresses everyone
• Cannot be ignored
• Must be embraced
• Is clearly defined
• Is a journey

WORDS *of* WISDOM

Change is challenging. It requires energy and commitment and can be ignored only at great personal expense. Accepting the change is the first step to successfully applying it to your own life.

~

The role of the leader is to translate changes to the staff, to find the meaning in the changes, and to get support and investment in those activities that facilitate the necessary changes. The two arenas for real change are form and behavior. Both must be altered in some measure to accommodate and implement change.

But what changes are real and enduring? How do we distinguish between the faddish and fashionable changes and the real, sustainable changes? (See Box 1-1.) Because of the amount of work required to implement any change, there simply is not the time or energy to spend on responses that are not meaningful.

SUSTAINING CHANGE

One of the primary roles of a leader is to discern the difference between what is short term and what is permanent. Managing work effort, which moves between responding to appropriate changes and implementing structure and process related to these changes, is a challenging activity at best. Leaders need the assurance that the path on which they have embarked will lead them to a more desirable state, resulting in the enhancement of work and the improvement of life. If this path accomplishes neither, the stakeholders in the change effort will lose interest in doing anything to promote possible change events.

For change to be clearly seen, it is important to have the proper frame of reference. In a change as significant as that which we are currently experiencing, we cannot use the context for viewing this change in the same way we have in the past. This change is broader and deeper than that which we have experienced previously, and our vision of the change is not adequate to see it appropriately (Box 1-2).

A NEW WAY OF SEEING

Our experience and insights tell us how what we see now compares to what and how we have seen things in the past. Our experiences validate what we are currently seeing and help us find meaning in it. However, we often see things for which our experience is inadequate to translate because what we see differs greatly from what we know; there is not sufficient context to help us translate what we see with any meaning. This scenario creates chaos as we try to sort out what we are seeing and search for some way to connect with it and find meaning in it.

TOWARD A NEW AGE

We are leaving the Industrial Age and moving toward an age that is still unclear to us but continues unfolding before us. Embedded in the journey to the new age are some very interesting circumstances.

It is difficult to embrace an age of change. Such an age confronts our sensibilities and threatens our stability. Our values, ways of knowing, experience, and belief systems were developed in the age we are leaving, and the journey is threatening.

Imagine what it means to leave a place that you know well, have grown up in, and have learned all of its intricacies, intimacies, and idiosyncrasies. Think about how it feels to have all of your values assaulted, experiences challenged, and knowledge diminished. This is what is contained within the context of an age change.

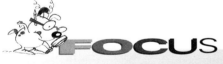

FOCUS

Embracing Change

- *Read the signposts.*
- *Assess your own response.*
- *Ask questions about what is happening.*
- *Read the journals and newspapers.*
- *Watch what others are doing.*
- *Talk it over with others.*
- *Keep an eye on how your work is changing.*
- *Get involved with the change makers.*
- *List your own strengths and needs.*
- *Rest and stay motivated.*

BOX 1-2

Change Is
1. Sociopolitical
2. Economic
3. Technical

Leaders must distinguish between what is real, sustainable change and what is simply faddish.

WORDS *of* WISDOM

The experience of transformation is like leaving home and living on your own for the first time. The world is the same but everything that tells you about it is now different and requires a response that no one else can provide for you. It is all about you now!

WORDS *of* WISDOM

The best way to make change work for us is to know as much about it as we can. We can do this by looking for all the indicators of change in the circumstances around us and applying the changes within that context. If it does not fit, we either must change what we are doing or examine the change more closely.

- *Technology has significantly altered our work, our lives, and our experiences.*
- *Communication systems have created a global community and have internationalized much of what was once local or national in design and function.*
- *Boundaries do not mean much anymore. The information infrastructure of society has contributed to the creation of a boundaryless world.*
- *Information is now the medium of exchange in a knowledgeable world. People with the right information can do anything they need to do anywhere it needs to be done.*
- *Building the information infrastructure will be the defining work of the next two decades. Organizations and systems will be radically moved from their identification with bricks and mortar structures to information-based structures.*
- *Workers are as important to the future as any other factor. Human capital is the growing essential medium of success for the future of enterprise on the global stage.*

READY FOR A JOURNEY

The challenge of change is to be able to engage the process of change at the right time and to understand the change as it confronts us. Furthermore, change requires a willingness to engage it in ways that bring sense and meaning to our experience.

During an age change, finding sense in the change is complicated because the change does not look like anything with which we are familiar. We are confronted with new content, character, and context. The emergence of the new age challenges what we know and have accepted as right and appropriate. Indeed, this new age requires us to see differently if we are to find the real meaning and impact of the change on our lives.

In this age change several significant issues have a major impact on our future.

The journey to a new age will certainly be exciting. It will also be traumatic.

THROUGH THE LOOKING GLASS

On the edge of a new age there is as much to be gained as there is to be lost. Since all of us were born in the Industrial Age, the journey into the new age will be challenging and "noisy."

All of our conceptual, formative, developmental, and experiential processes developed in the age that we are leaving. The challenge here is more than taking *the journey* into a new age. Indeed, much of how we see the journey, give it form, name its characteristics, and identify our role depends specifically on how we construct our response.

Much of what is emerging in this new age represents a way of thinking and knowing that fundamentally differs from past experiences. As stated previously, our greatest challenge is to be able to reflect the characteristics of the new age, not with what we know of the past, but with what we are willing and able to see in the emerging context. A number of strategies will be necessary to make this shift into what is essentially a new reality.

- Recognize that what we have experienced in the Industrial Age is no longer sufficient to the search for meaning in the new age.

- Being available to the changes is more important than being able to clearly define them. This means seeing the change in its own context rather than one we would create out of past experience.
- Continuously re-examining our perceptions, preconceived notions, and biases as an increasing weight of evidence calls us to a different place from that which we currently occupy.
- Embracing the challenge of the chaos in thinking and applying change, knowing that we are constructing the journey as we go and evaluating it in light of the outcomes we achieve.
- Disattaching ourselves from job content or processes as evidence suggests a need for altering them. Better defining ourselves by virtue of the outcomes achieved unbinds our blind identification to activity.
- Increasingly engaging other stakeholders in the dialogue of change. Sustainability will demand collective commitment and action from those who must give the new age form and function.

MOURNING THE LOSS

A shift of this significance cannot unfold without a great deal of conflict, uncertainty, and personal discomfort. On an almost daily basis, newspapers report on issues resulting from this shift: loss of jobs, mergers of well known institutions, economic and fiscal pressures, changes in social mores, and increase in cultural diversity, to name a few.

Furthermore, going to work brings no relief; indeed, it increases the stress. The fear that comes from anticipating the changes in the workplace and uncertainty about the future of the job creates a tension that is palpable. Not knowing is more difficult than implementing a change one already knows. The stability of the job and the content of work in the past could be counted on as a constant that provided some sense of permanence. With work redesign and restructuring, everyone is now thrown into a cauldron of changing relationships, new roles and functions, and the challenge of more change yet to come.

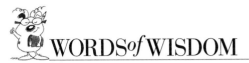

WORDS*of*WISDOM

We cannot make change without making noise. Change is not a quiet experience!

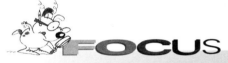

FOCUS

Necessary Losses

- *Old rituals*
- *Past routines*
- *Functions*
- *Position*
- *Job*
- *External security*
- *Location*
- *Permanence*
- *Certainty*
- *Guarantees*

Much of what is unfolding is an essential shift to a new reality. The chaos of these changes serves a real purpose. While this purpose is not terribly comforting, it is necessary. The chaos that exists in the moment between the "old" and the "new" serves to unbundle our attachment to what we are leaving. It creates a critical "noise" in the system that does not allow us to stay where we are. In some ways it forces us to confront the essential need for the change and our response to it. The key position between making the change and not moving creates the conditions that make action necessary. Sustainable action responds tightly to the change event. Nonsustainable response reacts to the change and contests its legitimacy and its impact on each of us. Reaction does not stop the change; rather, it simply delays our response to it.

People will hold on to what needs to be changed or will continue to revisit it if there is not sufficient time spent enumerating the losses embedded in the change and mourning the passing of practices, experiences, and relationships that exemplified the previous set of circumstances. Leaders must allow the staff and each other the time and space necessary to honor and mourn the loss if people are in any way to engage the changes they need to make without the encumbrances of yesterday.

Although mourning the passing of rituals and routines must be allowed, we cannot and should not mourn forever. The worst thing that could happen in the change journey is to become stuck in the passing and mourning of yesterday's experiences. A defined set of activities and a clear delineation of the time spent with loss is necessary (Box 1-3). Just as necessary is the need to move on at the appointed time. There must be a defined time established for that mourning period. Knowing the rules of passing is important to the stakeholders so that all can understand the expectation to work toward the appropriate response to the necessary changes.

MAKING SENSE OF THE FUTURE

People are much more willing to make a change if they can understand what that change means to them. Meaning is critical to positive response

---

BOX **1-3**

Letting Go

- Spend time with the change; get to understand it.
- Talk about what the change requires and what will happen.
- Personalize the change; make it mean something to you.
- Engage in a symbolic process that mourns the loss and allows it to pass.
- Let the old process go and close the door on it so you can focus on the new process and behaviors.

to change. The important role for a leader is to be able to translate the circumstances and conditions driving change in a language that can be understood by those who must undertake it (Team Tip 1-1).

The challenge for all agents in communicating change is their own understanding of it. All too often they struggle with sorting out what the change means and how it will impact them and their role. One of the characteristics of a good leader is the ability to manage personal uncertainty even while helping others deal with change. Translating, interpreting, and discussing the changes and challenges with staff members strengthen the relationship with and support of the staff and further refine everyone's understanding of the changes and their willingness to confront these changes together.

This notion of collective relationship is essential to the appropriate and sustainable response to change. Leadership must always know that even more important than clarity about the future is the willingness to be present to each other and to gather and offer mutual, individual, and collective support as people move together through the challenge of change.

In health care some specific changes are radically altering health service structures for the foreseeable future. The focus of this book is not to discuss these changes in great detail, but it is important to know what they are:

- Managed care is requiring all health services to be sensitive to the cost of providing services and to manage resources more effectively.

- Contracting for patients (managed lives) allows providers to know their patients before they serve them and to match services more closely to the needs of those served.

- Prepaying for services now requires that providers make better choices with patients about what services are provided and when and where these services should be offered. Knowing your patients (subscribers) means serving them before they become sick, thereby reducing both cost and intensity of service.

- Hospitals will no longer be the center of health care activity and will continue to decrease their numbers of beds. Indeed, the number of hospitals will decline.

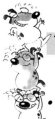

TEAMTIP   1.1

Leader's Role in Communicating Change

- Make sure you understand the change.
- Clarify any ambiguous elements before communicating with staff members.
- Make the change simple to understand.
- Share the change with staff members as soon as possible.
- Be frank and honest; no secrets allowed.
- Raise issues and concerns regarding the change and confront these issues at the outset.
- Communicate more information as you know it; do not hold back.

Be clear that the information you share about a change is accurate. Staff members hear so many rumors that they become uncertain. They need the assurance that what they respond to is correct and meaningful.

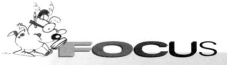

Have a Commitment to Experimentation

- Be open to explore new ways of thinking about work.
- Be willing to challenge current activities.
- Engage in dialogue with others about how different activities might work.
- Test new approaches and techniques to clinical activities.
- Evaluate outcomes of new processes to determine what works and what does not.

- Alternative, decentralized, portable service models will be created to better serve people where they work and live.
- Building the continuum of care for subscribers will require growing alliances, partnerships, and networks of services configured along the continuum to intersect with each other and patients in a more flexible, fluid, and comprehensive manner.
- Integration of service structures around patients will alter forever the design of services and systems and throw professionals and other providers together to sort out a new relationship built around the patient along the continuum of services.
- All people in health care will be required to change.

Clearly, significant changes are ahead in health service provision. In almost every conceivable way the system is changing around every role. In addition to the age change and the relentless forces of technology pushing at our backs, newer models of relationships and services are being constructed. Experimentation and innovation demand stretching and risking; testing newer approaches, models, structures, and relationships; and calling staff members to test what they do not yet fully comprehend. These are the circumstances of the time.

NO LONGER DOING MORE WITH LESS

How many times have we heard ourselves say that we must learn to do more with less? Too often we have said it to others when we did not have sufficient answers to their legitimate questions. Of course, it is not possible to do more with less forever. Given enough time, we would only end up do nothing with nothing.

As we move inexorably into a new age for work and health care, we will need to act differently. Indeed, we must fundamentally change what most of us are doing. It is no longer appropriate to simply continue to do work without carefully examining what the work is and what its impact is on achieving desirable and sustainable outcomes.

New circumstances and conditions call for new behaviors and expecta-

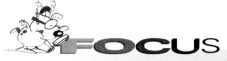

New Age for Health Care

These times call for a change in vision. The problem is that the context for the vision can often reflect what we understand of the "old ways" of seeing. The leader must try to visualize through "new eyes," looking from the perspective of the world into which we are moving. We will need:

- *Accurate information*
- *Proper tools*
- *An open mind*
- *Every role is subject to change. The leader must get all people to address their own needs in the change.*

What is different about the expectations for service, and how do these expectations affect what I do?

What is different in the environment of my work, and what response is it demanding of me?

What is the fit between what I am and have to offer and the changing demands on me as health service changes?

What do I need to learn to adapt or incorporate into my practice or work to better meet the emerging demands?

How have I personalized the changes to make sure I am aware of my responses, challenges, and need to change?

tions. A changing approach for providing services calls each of us to ask a different set of questions about who we are and the work we do.

The real "noise" of change is that it is always upon us and confronts us at times we may think are inappropriate or when we are unprepared for its effect on us. We are reminded that change is the only constant in the uni-

TEAM**TIP**   1.2

Making a Difference

People want to make a difference with their lives. This implies having meaning in the work they do. The leader should make sure to:

- *Tell the truth about the change.*
- *Help people build the change into their work.*
- *Show how the change is better or different.*
- *Allow people to discover the best way to apply the change.*

Remember that the care provider is interested in the impact of change on the patient and patient care. Ultimately the provider wants to do good work. Anything that appears to impede the ability to provide good service will run into serious trouble in its implementation. Opportunities to sabotage the process are automatic if the change agent does not give solid evidence that the change will not hurt patient care.

verse, and one of the questions change does not ask (because there is no answer) is whether we like it or not. Whether or not we like the change will not alter it or make it go away. Change is the eternal wind of the universe, chaos is its music, and transformation its song.

Finding meaning in our work requires not getting caught up in tasks and functions. Work is not tied into *what* we do but what we *achieve* (Team Tip 1-2). The outcome of our work is the final measure of its viability. If we are busy with many things and yet there is little evidence of impact or value, what does it matter how busy we are? "Busyness" does not in itself lend anything meaningful or desirable to our work.

If we are not busy with those things that make a difference and lead to some preferable result, where is the value in our work? Holding on to functions and activities that do not lead us to where we need to go, or result in what we thought we expected, keeps each of us on an activity treadmill—running hard but going nowhere.

Meaning in what we do is found in the connection between our activity and the purposes and outcomes to which that action is directed. The tightness of fit between what we do and what we achieve is the highest measure of effectiveness. In health care we increasingly see the need for a clear delineation between the work of health professions and the attainment of some desirable and sustainable outcome for those we serve. Today we need to have a more sustainable and cost-effective impact. This often means doing our work earlier in our relationship with the patient and doing things differently at that earlier point of service.

This earlier and different interaction with the patient will facilitate reduced cost and intensity, and reduced bed-based service, thereby keeping the patient from using hospital and high-intensity interventions to the fullest extent possible. That is not possible without changing what we do and how we do it. Our outcomes now change processes, activities, and functions. Without overstating this truth, outcomes change all we do and cause us to think critically about how we contribute to this emerging frame of reference for providing health care services.

TEAMS ARE EVERYTHING

In the emerging continuum of care, teams will be the essential unit of service (Box 1-4). Horizontal connections between providers and patients is the defining model for the future of health care services. The membership and construction of teams becomes the critical work of the organization.

In team-based pursuits, the models for service and organization radically change. No longer can the system be designed in a way that does not focus energies on the point-of-service and the primary relationship with those whom the system serves.

Team-based approaches conflict with almost everything that currently reflects the structure and relationships in hospitals and other components of the health care system. Several components of the system will have to be removed or "deconstructed" because they impede the creation of sustainable structures and relationships around the point-of-service in health care.

Clinical departments and discipline-specific structures prevent the formation of essential horizontal relationships between the professionals in a way that can more effectively serve the consumer.

Physicians, historically outside the cycle of relationships within the service system, have had no clearly enumerated accountability for outcomes and cost-effective performance.

Each of the disciplines have specific service standards and practices that have little relationship to each other. Each has a piece of the patient in the past; there has been little evidence of their interface with each other.

Organizational measures of performance and reward have always been individualized. As a result, these measures focus on the individual's work rather than value the integration of work activities between providers, all of whom offer some service to the patient.

In the past, no relationship between the rewards attached to positions and the outcomes of work or the impact on clinical results tied directly to the patient. No connection exists between what people do and what they are paid.

Organizations and their managers have acted primarily like parents in relationship to their staff members, thereby creating systems code-

BOX **1-4**

Teams: The Basic Unit of Service

The individual is no longer the basic unit of work; the team is. Individuals now must focus on building their relationships within the context of the team. It is the team that is the strongest work bond in the organization. Team members must:

- Know their work
- Know their partners
- Know their processes
- Know their outcome

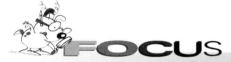

Organizations must attach rewards to performance in the future. There is simply no justification for paying for roles whose work outcomes are unknown. In the future rewards will reflect:

- Competence
- Performance
- Relationships
- Outcomes
- Value

Staff will make more decisions at the point-of-service in the future. The leader will need to make sure that staff members have the information and resources necessary to make the right decision the first time. Resource competency is no longer the strict province of the manager. Every member of the system has some accountability for the stewardship and use of resources.

pendency, subordinacy, and the resultant nonownership in workers regarding the value or productivity of their efforts. Simply inviting participation does not create ownership or investment in the worker. A shift in the locus of control does just that.

The design of a management chart and table of organization does not support the development and creation of an integrated, team-based, interdisciplinary service model. Moving decisions into the team's hands will accomplish this, but the losses to administration and management often impede or slow the process. Staff members are busy holding on to what they did in the past model of illness care. Now that the opportunity to expand roles, shift function, and advance accountability is available, staff members often object to the loss of ritual and routine that increasingly have no role or value in the emerging paradigm of health service.

The effort to configure the organization around the point of service and to facilitate the formation and effectiveness of teams is indeed challenging work. No one is left unaddressed in these efforts to create new relationships and interactions. The demand is to understand the character of change and the emerging context for health care in a subscriber-based, price-capitated continuum of care.

The traditional, vertically integrated organizational design for health systems is quickly dissipating in importance and being replaced throughout by the construction of a horizontally linked service continuum that represents the range of stakeholders and providers who configure their efforts and relationships around the service population that reflects the community served by the health system.

PRINCIPLES FOR A NEW AGE

Moving into a new paradigm for health care means discerning the essential principles that underpin the purpose and meaning of health care. The principles that once characterized the age out of which we are moving are now diminishing and shifting to a new set of foundations upon which society is being transformed.

For successful change to occur, these emerging principles must be clearly enumerated and take their rightful place as the foundation of the changes that will be built on them. There are four principles of the new age: partnership, equity, accountability, and ownership.

Partnership

Every where one looks the evidence of partnership in the global community abounds. Mergers, acquisitions, alliances, and networks are all terms synonymous with partnership. As the global community becomes more integrated and whole regions move into boundaryless configurations, the characteristics of partnership become increasingly more evident and important to the understanding and application of change.

In a partner-driven paradigm, it is important to recognize that the content, character, and relationships in work radically change. Just as every other component of society is altered, so too is the workplace. Partnership does not occur without effort, rather partnerships must be created. They demand a mutual value that drives the players into the relationship and requires work to define the essential characteristics of the partnership.

Partnership does not simply occur. It requires a mutual purpose, insight to the content of the partnership, and value each member will obtain from the relationship. All partnerships are negotiated and renegotiated over the life of the agreement. Each member has a unique value that he or she brings to the partnership, which must be carefully articulated and expressed within the context of the value added to the partnership.

Each member of a partnership believes that something of value can be obtained by joining efforts with others. The value of the partnership must extend beyond the value any one person can accomplish alone. Partnership is an equity-based relationship, which depends on the understanding between each member that the contribution each person makes is essential to the integrity of the partnership. This notion of value and contribution forms the foundation for sustainable partnerships.

A reason to enter into partnership and a purpose that brings meaning to

Almost everything in the new age exemplifies partnership. We are living in a boundaryless world where the information infrastructure connects and links all entities. Seamlessness and integration are the foundations of design for the workplace of the future.

Partnership is more than a connection. It is dynamic. It is present in the activities of all systems as they attempt to construct a sustainable format within which they can thrive. All the links necessary are addressed to ensure that the right connections are in place to ensure meaning and value.

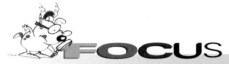

the relationship must always be present. Each member must see an advanced or improved value or circumstance through entering into the partnership. This implies that the rewards of partnership are as clear as the work, and that the price paid for the construction of partnership is found in its fruits and rewards.

Partnership also demands a clarity and honesty of interaction so that each member is able and free to bring up issues and concerns regarding the character of the partnership. A partnership is always a work in progress. Continual renegotiation, dialogue, changing circumstances and positions, and new opportunities' needs are forever rising out of the expression and work of the partnership, thereby requiring continual discourse and renewal.

Partnership changes everything for an individual. Where it was once possible to make decisions without the consideration of others, this is not possible with partners. A partnership is often characterized as another person or structure that emerged at the creation of the "third entity" called partnership. Being dynamic rather than an event, partnership demands continual attention and service. Each of the leaders of the partnership will continually reassess and shift the conditions of the partnership, in the effort to advance or improve the conditions and circumstances affecting the viability of the partnership.

The new language of health care has embedded in it the implications for the formation of a wide variety of partnerships. Many of these more local partnerships must converge to assume a larger and more powerful work relationship. These networks, alliances, integrations, and mergers are all different ways of expressing the idea and practice of partnership. As is apparent, partnerships are becoming the foundation for many of the new health care models emerging in response to the demand for a more effective health system.

The notion of partnership moves toward the point-of-service. As patient-based approaches become the norm in designing patient care services, there is increasing need for partnership between providers and with patients. To apply this notion would unbundle a range of current practices and all the hostilities around independent and discipline-driven loci of control. Emphasis on the various parts of an organization at the expense of the whole is no longer tenable, nor can it support the system's ability to thrive. Many of the patterns of behavior that have emerged out of historical compartmentalism are now subject to great suspicion and may fall deeper within the context of the current shifts in the health care system. These circumstances create the conditions for partnership and form the foundations for requiring it.

Because the health care system has not operated within the constructs of partnership in the past, there will be much work to do. Creating the clinical continuum necessitates a foundation in relationship at a level of connectedness and intensity not previously experienced. Teams of clinical providers become stakeholders in the process and must connect their energies and work together to produce standards, protocols, quality measures, and outcome determinations that can only be achieved through their mutual efforts. Partnership, rather than a luxury, becomes a requisite for sustainable health services for the future.

Equity

If the value of each person contributing to the relationship is not noted a lasting relationship cannot form. Equity is the measure of value attached to the contribution of each of the members of a relationship. In equity we assume that value is attached to the contribution of each player to a team or partnership and that this activity lends value to the work of the group. In these circumstances every member of the group is expected to recognize this and incorporate it into his or her behavior and expressions of membership and work.

There is nothing more denigrating to the integrity of the group than to diminish the value of any one member through the application of ascendant behaviors or critical judgments between individual members and others in the group. Also, leveling, or creating a hierarchy of importance around the various contributions of members, diminishes the relationships essential to maintain the integrity of the group.

Partnership demands that there be a sense of equality between the players. Each person contributes something of value to the relationship and needs to be honored for that contribution. Also, each partner's expectations include the right to receive full value from the relationship. Each member must give fully to the work of the partnership to advance the partnership and ensure it produces desired outcomes.

Equity is not equality; it is instead about value. At work, relationships must give evidence of their contribution to the purposes of the system to have any value.

Equity as a value demands that each essential contribution be viewed as an important part of the work of the whole. There should be a realization that the group's work is the aggregation of the efforts of all its members and that sustainability is impossible without the convergence of the efforts of everyone upon whom the outcome depends. The effectiveness of the team depends on this understanding. There is nothing that destroys teams and their effectiveness more than the pettiness and inequity of members in their dealings with each other. Equity is an essential constituent of every team and is facilitated through respect for each other's roles and the clarity of the contribution each one makes. Building that into the function of teams creates a firm foundation upon which to build effectiveness.

Accountability

Personal accountability is becoming increasingly important to the effectiveness of achieving clinical outcomes in any health setting. As focusing on the outcome accelerates, the contribution to the outcome of each role in the system becomes vital. Knowing what that contribution is and how it fits with contributions of others is a significant activity of work groups today. Much work has been done on the issue of quality and outcome. The importance of defining the relationship of processes to outcomes for the sustainability of meaningful work activities is becoming clearer. The activities of work have no meaning in their performance unless that performance achieves some valued result; simply performing work has no value if that performance does not tightly fit with the outcomes toward which it is directed.

This fit between process and outcome, so prevalent in workplaces today, has created a need to become fully aware of the content of work and the contribution of each job in relationship to the expectations and outcomes to which they are directed. Never has so much focused on streamlining the fit between roles and their outcomes than has occurred in the past decade. Increasingly, the emphasis has been on defining the specific contribution to the outcome each role makes and determining just how "tight" is the connection between the two. This has been especially problematic for

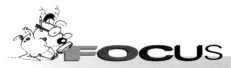

Accountability is:
- *Outcome driven*
- *Always expressed at the personal level*
- *Never delegated*
- *Competency based*
- *Evaluated with clear consequences*
- *Generated from the point-of-service*

many workers because it means focusing more intently on the content of their work and facing the conflict that comes from decisions that require the elimination of many roles and functions in an organization.

Accountability focuses on defining the outcomes of a role and giving evidence of having obtained the related outcomes. Different from responsibility, accountability focuses on what is produced or results as the measure of efficacy rather than simply on the content of the job. Work content and results must have a tight fit to justify the existence of a role and find value in it. Sustainable roles are those where the outcomes continually adjust or refine the expectation for function and performance. Within this frame of reference accountability takes its meaning and derives its value. An accountable person is one who sees work from the perspective of achievement and value. An accountable individual owns the obligation for performance and is committed to the measurement and application of functions, tasks, and activities in light of the outcomes to which they are directed (Box 1-5). The future of work includes the understanding that accountability is a requisite of every position and will be the foundation of the measures of performance for some time to come.

Ownership

In the new age the notion of work and workplace relationships, often expressed in terms of superior-subordinate, master-servant, employer-employee, and parent-child, really have little sustainable value for any one. The notion that the workplace is the "playpen" of the owners of the means of work is no longer valid. Data have proven that such vertical and parental notions of work and performance are not sustainable.

This reality has created a new approach to understanding work and the worker at every place work is done. The age change has brought with it an understanding of the value of work and its relationship to the whole enterprise. In systems views of work essentially two sources of real value in the organization exist: financial capital and human capital. Respect, integration, and appreciation of both are essential to create the conditions necessary to ensure an enterprise's sustainability.

BOX **1-5**

Individual Accountability

My accountability:
- I have to show that my work has value.
- I need to relate well with my peers.
- What I do is a part of the whole—it must fit.
- If I do not perform, there are consequences to us all.
- I need feedback to ensure that my team and I have a mutual understanding of my role.
- We must evaluate often what we are doing to ensure it still has value.

Ownership is essential to effective and sustainable outcomes. For too long the sense of ownership has been missing from the work of those at the point-of-service and was held by those who managed. Good and sustainable service outcomes are rarely achieved by managers. Instead those who own the work they do ensure continuing effectiveness and lasting quality.

In a systems view, all the participants in an enterprise are essential to its success, or they should not be there. Ownership assumes that stakeholders exist at every place in the organization. Each player in a system has a stake in the success of the work of the system. Each person makes a contribution that either adds to or diminishes the value of the system. Every person must see themselves within the context of contribution and not simply as the recipient of employment. This means moving beyond the framework of a job orientation, a passive connection to work that is no longer viable. More investment and connection is needed in knowledge-driven organizations than was evidenced in the past. The principle of ownership takes its form from this frame of reference.

A part of the expectations for team-based processes is that each team member be fully invested in the work of the team and the relationship between its members. This investment must reflect a sense of ownership between each of the participants of their contribution to the work and effectiveness of the team. This level of commitment reflects the ownership necessary to build a collective energy directed toward the achievement of mutual outcomes.

The need for increasing a sense of ownership in the workplace is perhaps the most challenging activity of the time. When downsizing and reconfiguring organizations to be more appropriately in line with their resources and effectiveness, the temptation for workers is to lose interest, diminish commitment, and segment into job saving and functionalism ("I'll just do *my* job"). The better strategy, however, is the opposite, that is, to join more intently on creating a better fit, increasing skills and value, and positioning fluidly for those new roles and expectations that emerge from the chaos of restructuring.

Ownership is exemplified by engaging in change and embracing the challenges that result in personal growth. No organization will be successful in the new age without the investment of the stakeholders, regardless of where they are located in the system.

There is no more valid notion of "My Job" any longer. All work depends on relationship and good "fit" between people and processes. In a system, the intersection of all roles becomes the foundation for ensuring that the mission and purposes get fulfilled every place work is done.

CHANGE AS A JOURNEY

The movement to committed and invested teams is not something that is accomplished or completed overnight. Indeed, it is a journey with many twists and turns and ups and downs along the way. In each stage of building team relationships there are challenges that can facilitate or strain the development of a team consciousness.

Everyone needs supplemental support and information along the way to effective relationship building and team formation. The strength of teams and their success depends on the team's attention to its own needs for growth and development. Many tools can supply information and support to each member as the team takes form and begins to function well together.

This TEAMbook is designed to render some encouragement and tools to the team builder in a health care environment. It is one of a number of "tool chests" that should be a part of the information base for team members and their facilitators.

Remember that the principles discussed above are the foundations upon which all team efforts are validated and evaluated. These principles serve as the baseline for measuring the constituents of the journey and the products of the work of team building. Sustainability in the organization will depend on how the processes of the team resonate with the principles that reflect the age change.

The leader must always experiment, challenge, test, and struggle to keep what works and discard what does not. There are many moments in building effective teams when the process either seems overwhelming or does not appear to be fruitful. This, too, is part of the dynamic of team building. Success takes time.

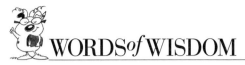

WORDS *of* WISDOM

The journey to a new health system means dismantling some of the old to make room for the new. What we need to bring with us from the past, we should bring. What we do not need, we should leave behind. Good leadership knows the difference between the two.

Bibliography

Alexander J, Zuckerman H, Pointer D: The challenges of governing integrated health systems, *Health Care Management Review* 20(4):69-81, 1995.

Ashkenas R et al: *The boundaryless organization,* San Francisco, Jossey-Bass, 1995.

Bartlett C, Ghoshal S: Changing the role of top management: beyond systems to people, *Harvard Business Review* 73(3):132-142, 1995.

Bergquist WJ, Betwee, Meuel D: *Building strategic relationships,* San Francisco, Jossey-Bass, 1995.

Brown M, McCool B: Health care systems: predictions for the future, *Healthcare Management Review* 15(3):87-94, 1990.

Cave D: Vertical integration models to prepare health systems for capitation, *Healthcare Management Review* 20(1): 26-39, 1995.

Channon J: Social architecture: can we design a new civilization, *World Business Academy Perspectives* (3):19-32, 1995.

Coile R: Transformation of American healthcare in the post reform era, *Healthcare Executive* 9(4):8-12, 1994.

DeWoody S, Price J: A systems approach to multidimensional critical paths, *Nursing Management* 25(11):47-51, 1994.

Doerge J, Hagenow N: Integrating care delivery, *Nursing Administration Quarterly* 20(2):42-48, 1996.

Eisler R: The hidden subtext for sustainable change, *World Business Academy Perspective* 9(3):45-58, 1995.

Gould J, DiBella A, Nevis E: Organizations as learning systems, *The Systems Thinker* 4(8):1-3, 1993.

Griffith J: Re-engineering healthcare: management systems for survivors, *Hospital & Health Services Administration* 39(4):23-35, 1994.

Griffith J: The infrastructure of integrated delivery systems, *Healthcare Executive* 10(3):12-17, 1995.

Hitchings K, Kinnemann M: A professional development model to foster change, *Seminars for Nurse Managers* 2(4):229-233, 1994.

Holland J: *Hidden order,* New York, Addison-Wesley, 1995.

Keidel R: *Seeing organizational patterns,* San Francisco, Berrett-Koehler, 1995.

Kim D: *Toward learning organizations,* Cambridge, Mass, Pegasus, 1992.

Kotter J: Leading change: why transformation efforts fail, *Harvard Business Review* 73(2):59-67, 1995.

MacDonald A: Integrating management of physician groups and hospitals, *Topics in Healthcare Financing* 20(4):48-54, 1994.

Macy J: Collective self interest-the holonic shift, *World Business Academy Perspectives* 9(1):19-22, 1995.

Manthey M: Delivery systems and practice models: a dynamic balance, 22(1):28-30, 1991.

Martin J: *The great transition: using the seven disciplines of enterprise engineering to align people, technology, and strategy,* St Louis, AMACOM Publications, 1996.

Moore J: *The death of competition,* New York, Harper Business, 1996.

Porter-O'Grady T: Building partnerships in health care: creating whole systems change, *Nursing & Healthcare,* 15(1):34-38, 1994.

Oshry B: *Seeing systems: unlocking the mysteries of organizational life,* San Francisco, Berrett-Koehler, 1995.

Porter-O'Grady T: A systems approach to managing change, *Seminars for Nurse Managers* 2(4):191-195, 1994.

Porter-O'Grady T, Krueger-Wilson, C: *The leadership revolution in healthcare: altering systems, changing behavior,* Gaithersburg, Md, Aspen Publishers, 1995.

Shortell S: Creating organized delivery systems: the barriers and facilitators, *Hospitals & Health Services Administration* 33(4):447-466, 1993.

Shortell S et al: *Remaking healthcare in America,* San Francisco, Jossey-Bass, 1996.

Snyder-Halpern R: Healthcare system innovation: a model for practice, *Advanced Nursing Practice Quarterly* 1(4):12-19, 1996.

Wheatley M: *A simpler way,* San Francisco, Berrett-Koehler, 1996.

Wilson T: *Innovative reward systems for the changing workplace,* New York, McGraw-Hill, 1995.

TOOLCHEST

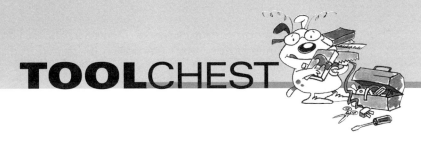

TOOL A: The Team Bill of Rights[*]

Each team must be free to do their work and exercise their judgment within the context of the authority given. Therefore teams have certain rights as well as responsibilities. These rights form the underpinnings for determining whether successful teams have been created and whether they are able to do their work.

The following rights are identified within the context of freedoms. Teams have a responsibility to undertake their activities successfully. Gifford and Elizabeth Pinchot* have identified several freedoms, in the open organizational system. Reflecting these freedoms, the following elements of the team bill of rights are created:

Freedom 1: The Right of Expression
All members of the team have the right to speak freely; to be able to communicate effectively in honest and truthful ways; and to be able to share frankly, truthfully, and openly the issues, perceptions, and concerns brought forth in team dialogue.

Freedom 2: The Right to Learn
All participants on a team have a right to grow, adjust to change, and become. Therefore they are able

*Pinchot G, Pinchot E: *The end of bureaucracy and the rise of the intelligent organization,* San Francisco, Berrett-Koehler, 1993.

to be involved in inquiry, access information, build knowledge, and expand their competence. As a result, they have the right to be curious and persistent, expand their awareness, seek successes, to enumerate failures, and continue to develop skills and ability and make learning a lifelong process.

Freedom 3: The Right to Work
Every member of an organizational team has the right to do the work of the team and fulfill their obligations as members of the team. Therefore they have the right to participate in projects and priorities to determine their level of contribution and apply their gifts and their skills as fully as possible. They have the right to own and apply the tools of their profession or work and to commit to worthwhile activities with the full range of their skills and efforts. Each team member has the right to act with courage and maintain integrity and to be a fully involved, participating member of the team.

Freedom 4: The Right of Enterprise
Each team member has a right to be influenced by the persons they serve, that is, the patients and customers who drive response to their work and interactions. Therefore they have a right to establish a way of exchanging relations, information,

and interaction with those they serve. They have an obligation to use the resources wisely and live within their means. They have an obligation to give fair measure of their work, have that work honored and consistently incorporated into the organization's goals and objectives, and participate in the rewards that would imply.

Freedom 5: The Right to Work as a Team Member

Every member of a system is a member of an organization. Membership-driven organizations operate differently from employee-constructed structures. Therefore every team member has a right to participate in decisions; work freely with teammates; participate in choosing those teammates; share joint ownership in the team processes; and be able to benefit from the rewards, opportunities, and outcomes of the team's work. Each member has a right to achieve the goals, make good decisions in participation with others, care for and support other teammates, and look for others to become teammates who are consistent with the character and expectations of the team.

Freedom 6: A Right to Be a Member of Community of Differences

Every member, regardless of their background, experience, frame of reference, and value system, has a right to full membership in the organization when they become a member. They have a right to a community of caring, of investment, of support—a group that is ethical and works well together in support of the purposes of the organization. They have a right to experience tolerance and nonprejudice. They have the obligation to balance self-interest against the common good and to work out the differences between the two. All members of

the community have a right to work toward worthwhile outcomes, use appropriate vision and values to construct them, and find support for their diversity and their contribution.

Freedom 7: Justice and the Rule of Law

Each individual has the right to experience due process to ensure that the judgment is fair and equitable and that they have been treated in balance by the support of their peers. The expectation is that all team members are law abiding and support the rules, standards, and practices in which they have all agreed to participate to establish good process and framework for work, and to be consistent, balance self-serving in a way that serves the issues of others, to avoid entitlement, and to seek opportunities to fight injustice and inequity wherever it may be found.

Freedom 8: Democratic Process

Each individual has the right to participate fully in the contribution of the team's outcomes. Self-management and self direction of the team within the boundaries established are appropriate for all team members. Every member has the right to participating and designing its relationship to the larger system and in the larger system support of it. Each member has an obligation to listen and to be heard; to learn and to be taught; to teach and to stand for the commitments, principles, and values to which the team has committed.

Freedom 9: The Freedom of Interrelationships

Each member of the team has the right to associate and aggregate with those who facilitate, encourage, or promulgate the purposes of the individual in the team, as well as to make choices with regard to those they associate with and how those associations will be built. They have the obligation and the freedom to honor and respect the commitments of each member of the team, to make their commitments appropriately and be wise in their application, to deliver one's commitments and honor the commitments made, to use time carefully and wisely, and to serve the larger community as a part of their commitment to the team.

Freedom 10: Limits on Systems Governance

Every system should support the activities of that which occurs at its point-of-service. Therefore the role of a system is to provide the support necessary to enhance the relationship between the provider and those served. Every individual should support the right of every member of the team in the system. Constitutional, policy, and structural limits are placed on inappropriate and unnecessary control of the individual. The governance structure is one that guides the system and creates a fit between all the components of the system, thereby ensuring that all come together to facilitate the work and the value of the system. The system's governance makes sure that the incentives and mandates of the system are fairly and equitably applied and continue to advance the work of each individual as well as the team. Planning and strategic work are expected to reflect farsightedness in a commitment to long-term sustainability, and all decisions should generate from the point-of-service and be supported by a system whose role is to see that the mission and purposes of the organization are fulfilled at every level of the system.

TOOL B : Change Mapping

Many changes are moving at a rapid pace through the health care system. The struggle for each individual is to be able to cope and keep up with the impact of change on the individual's work and the goals for their own work and career. To thrive in the new environment, each person must understand his or her relationship to work and the impact the relationship has on adapting to work. These questions relate to specific individual adaptation to the changes that affect job course and personal direction.

Goals of the Instrument

1. To ensure that individuals spend time looking at their roles, jobs, and careers.

2. To allow the individual to analyze past choice and future choice, and to see the fit between where they are and where they are going.
3. To help the individual understand the activities necessary to achieve personal goals.
4. To identify and assess the direction of the individual's career.
5. To develop a framework for actions that individuals might take to fulfill personal choices.

Instruction and Process

1. The facilitator outlines the general activities and the need to help individuals seek the difference between where they are and the goals that they attempt to achieve. Each indi-

vidual has a copy of this instrument and uses it for the framework for the questions at each table. Group size for this tool is as many as 25 individuals in groups of 4 to 6 members; the time required is 2 to 3 hours of group work.

2. Questions contained in this instrument are answered at each table by each individual at the table as fully and as completely as possible in about 15 to 20 minutes.

3. After completing the questions each group member shares with other group members the content of their personal career goals and issues based on the questions that they answered. This takes about 30 minutes of discussion time.

4. Discussion stops, and each individual outlines the specific demarcations of his or her career pathway from initiation to what may be considered important or defining moments in the work or career path. Each demarcation is identified on a sheet of paper and connected with a line that shows a continuation or road that links each demarcation with the other. The group then discusses the specific elements for 20 minutes.

5. Based on the discussion each individual identifies two to three elements of future choices that need to be made in his or her career, job, or work pathway. These choices serve as the foundation for the next level of dialogue in the group, which lasts about 20 minutes.

6. After the discussion, each member of the group identifies at least two action items that he or she will implement within the next year. Once an individual names these, he or she will share them with the group and commit to their implementation.

Career Development Pathway Questions

1. What specific event, circumstance, or condition stimulated you to select your current career pathway?

2. Where did you start your development and education for this career pathway?

3. Do you feel good about the choice you made? If not, what other choice would you have made?

4. Identify two significant events that validate the path you have taken.

5. In 5 year increments identify the specific role in your career you've had.

6. Where are you currently on your career path? Where has this path brought you?

These questions serve as the foundation upon which discussion begins and builds. Using the information gained in this foundation, the subsequent questions and activities of the team can be undertaken. Each participant should remember that the goal is to identify the next stages and activities in which he or she will contribute, and then begin to make judgments about where to move and what activity each person will need to undertake to achieve the career or role changes identified.

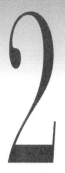

Working in a New World: Transforming the Organizational Structure

Innovation is a combination of brains and materials.
The more brains you have, the less material you need.
Charles Kettering

TRANSFORMING THE WORLD

The world is in the midst of major social transformation, one that extends to every element of our social experience, including the workplace. Although health care systems have come to this transformation later than other segments of our society (notably business), health care systems are now in the throes of dramatic shifts from the old, sickness-based system to a new focus on providing a health-based delivery system. This is not to suggest that the designs and structures currently underway will result in a truly health-based delivery system. However, the initial activities necessary to create a healthy society and health-based outcomes are beginning to emerge.

Much of the effort to move toward integrated health care includes creating seamless design, whole systems approaches, managed care, measures of quality care, outcome-driven evaluation, and a host of other related elements. Each of these are a sign of the shift in health care within a context similar to that of the business community. Although broad disagreement exists as to which strategies should be chosen to effectively change and improve the health care system, activities in that direction are well underway.

Just as processes are being shifted to meet new requirements, so are their supporting structures. Nothing will affect good process more than the appropriate structure that facilitates it. One of the major problems in much of today's redesigned activities is that they have the right process and the wrong structure.

BOX 2-1

Teams: The Foundation of Work

The basic unit of work for the foreseeable future is the team. This is a shift from focus on the work of the individual. The team is a more accurate foundation of work because:

- Outcomes depend on collective contribution.
- Relationship defines the distribution of work activities.
- Integration of work is necessary to sustainability.

As more health systems focus on their point-of-service as the primary focus of control for work, health systems will become more skilled in the movement to team-based integration for the design of clinical work.

TEAMS—THE BASIC UNIT OF WORK

Much of the research of the last 30 years has helped organizational leadership determine that the basic unit of work is the team rather than the individual (Box 2-1). Of course, individuals are important to the process of work, but the outcomes of work depend on the integration of the activities of many people. Therefore, while individuals are important in undertaking work process, the relationship between people is a greater measure of the products of work. The interaction and intersection between people in undertaking work becomes increasingly critical to the viability of the outcomes of that work.

The idea of organizing work within the context of team-based approaches is relatively new, radically altering the basic structure and relationship in most organizations around the world. Initially concepts of empowerment, team relationships, personal involvement, ownership, and stakeholdership were generated from the Scandinavian academic and business communities. These concepts have been adapted and studied throughout the world. A database of concepts supporting point-of-service and team-based approaches has driven leaders in the workplace to not only consider their inclusion in organizing and managing work, but also in building the fundamentals of the design of work, the organizational structure, management roles, and worker relationships around such concepts.

The reader might say at this point, "So what? It sounds rational and appropriate to recognize the value of the contribution of people to each other and to the work that they do together. What is so new about that?" Good question. While it is rational, the design of the workplace has been based on a different set of principles. The belief of the locus of control for workplaces rests in the hands of those who own the means of work, and productivity is a fundamental tenet of capitalism. We have begun to recognize in systems approaches and in quantum mechanics theory behind them that a broader notion of ownership and relationship is necessary to create sustainable circumstances for work.

The ownership model, hierarchical structure, vertical design, and parent/child relationships between management and staff are all examples of the old organizational beliefs about work and work relationships. None of those beliefs fits appropriately in a broader understanding of how systems work. More meaningful today are the notions of stakeholdership and ownership of work; the investment of all players in the mission, purposes, and outcomes of the enterprise; and the ability of each member of the system to contribute something meaningful to the work and its products within the system. Each of these realities creates an entirely new construct for the design of work, thus shifting the focus away from old command and control structures to more integrative models that recognize the value of contribution at all points in the organization.

Perhaps the single largest conflict in the move to a new organizational design is that which is exhibited as organizations change from centralized, hierarchical management-driven structures into more point-of-service, relational, and team-based structures (Box 2-2). The changes in behavior and style in relationship, expectation, roles, and intersection create a requirement for a dramatic shift in design of the organization and the behavior of its members. Most of the organizational change is generated within this effort, and this is where most of the difficulties arise in making new structures work.

THE ORGANIZATIONAL UNDERPINNINGS FOR TEAM-BASED APPROACHES

A movement to teams requires a major shift in understanding and belief. At every level of the organization, members of the system are required to establish a different set of roles and relationships with each other that reflect more equity-based approaches to the delivery of service, decision-making process, and interaction and relationship building.

In the old model of organization, the role of the manager was to plan, organize, lead, implement, control, and evaluate. (Is it coincidence that the first letter of each of the management roles spells "POLICE"?) These old delineations of management are no longer appropriate to the expectations for

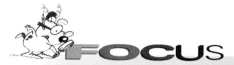

FOCUS

Team-based approaches demand a fuller understanding of systems models. Health professionals can no longer look at their own work outside the context of its impact on the work of others. Key players who must integrate their activities include:

- Nurses
- Physicians
- Pharmacists
- Therapists
- Technologists

BOX **2-2**

Changing the Control Systems

Movement to teams demands a change from vertical and hierarchical control systems to horizontal and team-based models. Some past requirements that must be discarded include:

- Centralized control systems
- Hierarchical management approaches
- Limited information support systems
- Standardized human resource practices
- Command and control governance and administrative processes

the new role of leader. The worker was primarily responsible for doing what was assigned, fulfilling the job description, and undertaking the job tasks and functions in the manner prescribed by the organization. This rather mindless, subordinated approach to delineating and doing work has in the past hundred years created a chasm between management and staff.

Problems in relationship, productivity, communication, and interactions necessary to support sustainable work outcomes have resulted from this ("us/them") behavioral pattern of work. Some major social institutions are in part the result of these work constructs. Unions, management-driven disciplinary processes, workers "job" orientation, noncreative worker functionalism, and worker isolation are all examples of the results of this kind of organizational construct. These constructions create the conditions that make it difficult to change worker relationships and behaviors. The dependencies evidenced in this kind of an organizational construct create conditions that, while dysfunctional, result in a level of comfort and apathy, as well as ritual and routine, which are difficult to overcome.

Different beliefs about work, worker relationship, accountability, outcomes, and so on, require a shift in thinking as well as an adjustment in behavior. Every member of the organization will undergo some specific personal adjustment in making this change work.

If team-based behaviors are to emerge, team constructs require both a different set of beliefs and different processes for implementing these beliefs. Much of the mistrust that exists in many organizations is the result of the environment that facilitates it. A shift in that environment itself breeds further mistrust, making it difficult for people to commit at the outset to a major change in the organizational structure and the work process. Critical work of team-based leadership, in part, is to build strategies to address what those specific changes will be.

All teams must be accountability based in their design and work. Teams must focus on outcomes if they are to fulfill their obligation to contribute to the success of the system.

THE WHOLE SYSTEM AS TEAM

To ensure success, all members of the organization must see themselves as part of a team. No one member can act unilaterally out of the context of his or her relationship to other members of the team. This creates a discipline that requires a different kind of interaction and communication strategies in the organizational system. It further requires a personal discipline with regard to behavior, role, and dialogue between the various components and people in the organization.

Disciplining one's behavior within the context of a broader set of relationships requires a change in the supporting structure. Not only does structure have to shift support for disciplined behavior, but so do the principles that guide it. Team-based behaviors exemplify the principles of partnership, equity, accountability, and ownership. For those to be expressed in the workplace, a commitment must be made throughout the system to the same ideals and processes regardless of where work is done (Team Tip 2-1). The orientation of the organization and its structure must be such that it supports that possibility (i.e., everyone committed to the same goals) and exemplifies the organization's consistent commitment and practices based on the principles that drive it. Several components of the change process drive the organization to the principles of partnership, equity, accountability, and ownership. These exemplary components are basic requisites in the new organizational system. They must be clearly defined to provide a foundation for the change in both structure and behavior.

Components of the Change Process

Patient-service focus

All organizations should be designed to support the activities that go on as point-of-productivity or point-of-service. In health care, patient care is the central functional activity of the organization. Focusing on the consumer of services, whether identified as the subscriber, patient, client, or partner, is the fundamental component of the design of any system. This point-of-service structuring is critical to the integrity and sustainability of any health system.

TEAMTIP   2.1

Team Commitment to Change
In the course of doing their work, staff members must be prepared to do the following two things differently from the past:
- *Integrate the decisions each person makes with the goals of the team.*
- *Incorporate the systems objectives with the outcomes of clinical work.*

Outcomes drive everything. If there are no sustainable results there is no work.

Empowerment means that people have the power necessary to do the work for which they are accountable. We cannot expect people to sustain that over which they have no power!

Mission drives everything, from the boardroom to the patient's bedside. All activities in the system must reflect the mission.

Health is the outcome

In the past, institutions providing health service in the United States focused on sickness and its treatment. A much broader context now exists for the provision of health services. Support for the achievement of the community's health and that of its members now is a major part of the mission and functional framework for the health system.

Structure always supports function

The design of an organization always should relate specifically to its purposes and the work it does. Partnership between members of the health care organization and the community it serves requires a different configuration and organizational design. Structuring to support the point-of-service and building around it, creating only as much structure as needed to maintain the organization's integrity and effectiveness, is a critical part of transforming the health care system.

Empower the point-of-service

To achieve effectiveness, good decision making must be expressed and right outcomes must be obtained. Those who are accountable for producing the outcomes must be free to do what is necessary to achieve good results. Every component of the organization should be structured and designed to support the achievement of results in the places where the work that drives those results is performed.

Configure around mission

Development and maintenance of a mission is not the sole work of the governance leadership of an organization. Mission provides the framework for the purposes and objectives of all work in a system. If a system is to be successful, all members must have some ownership of the mission. Configuring around mission, incorporating it into all activities and levels of work, and exemplifying it in the production of clinical and service outcomes are critical to the validation of the meaning and purpose of an organization. Every member of the system must at some level have ownership of the mission, and mission should be integrated into the plans and activities of every player in the system.

Build a seamless service continuum

Creating and facilitating health is not an event, but a continuous process that addresses the needs of consumers at different points along their health care journey. Connecting and linking components of the system in a meaningful way is the fundamental work of providing a focus on health care and achieving good health-based results. The relationship between and among providers, patients, and community is continuous in the health care system. This continuous, dynamic intersection of players in a cycle of changing demands, relationships, processes, and activities is a part of a healthy, viable health care system. A fundamental need of an effective, integrated health care system is to create a structure to support that dynamic relationship and facilitate its sustainability.

Ensure team effectiveness

If sustainable products of work are achieved through the critical intersection between people and process in a system, leadership must always focus on ensuring the integrity and effectiveness of those relationships and processes. Team-based approaches to service delivery recognize the inherent relatedness between all provider, patient, and community roles in a health system. Building a consistent, well designed, fluid, team-based system for service delivery is one of the critical elements of the work and value of an organization.

Create the learning organization

Organizations, like the people who make them up, are continuously changing and adjusting to the context and realities that form the framework for their services. Change is a universal constant. The ability to adjust and to fluidly respond to change is a critical condition for long-term

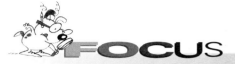

The team is the central component of the design of structure. Teams essentially:

- Sit at the center of the organizational structure
- Make 90% of the decisions about service
- Are the system's primary contact with the patient
- Design and control the patient's clinical path
- Measure and control the quality of service provided

Today, all organizations are centers of learning. In the changing health care environment everything is being shifted and altered, thereby requiring the commitment of everyone from board chair to housekeeper to become learners on the journey toward transformation.

viability in any system. The ability of the members to implement changes, to adjust their own roles and practices, and to expand their knowledge base are all fundamental to the integrity and viability of any service system. Therefore building a system must account for the need to be continuously aware of the learning dynamic and the understanding that every participant in the system is a learner. The very construction of the system must incorporate the understanding that it is forever adapting and adjusting.

Keep the centrality of principle

Principles exemplify, in an intelligible way, action founded in meaning. Principles reflect the meaning to which people attach their thoughts, values, and activities. They form the anchor that continually "calls back" the individual to reflect on that foundation upon which all thought, value, and activity take form. Principles provide the conceptual and lived foundations out of which come the urge to act and the resultant activities. Principles become the core of evaluating efficacy, effectiveness, and meaning of thought and action.

Principle drives everything. Principle-centered organizations require every member to find his or her work centered on the core principles that define the system.

In health systems, the principles of partnership, equity, accountability, and ownership lie at the core of all team efforts. Every team, if it is effective and fulfilling the purposes of the organization, should reflect on the principles that form its foundation. The notion of partnership should be a fundamental part of the thinking of each member of the team. Each member has a contribution to make and is obliged to make that contribution to fully participate in the activities of the team. This is a sign of the presence of equity. Accountability is exemplified in the evidence of staff members' fulfillment above performance and expectation requirements in their roles as negotiated between and among members of the team. Accountability exemplifies the level of personal investment and commitment as a member of the team to the purposes, work, and activities of the team. Ownership is exemplified in the sense that each member of a team is a stakeholder in the enterprise, holds some investment in its value and continuance, and has a commitment not only to personal activities but to helping the team and the system it supports thrive.

The four principles of the new age-partnership, equity, ownership, and accountability-are central to the correct structuring of the system. They serve as the template on which every element of redesign can be evaluated and every clinical process can be measured.

Principles can be used as a part of the evaluative process to determine whether teams and individuals have acted consistently with the expectations they have with, for, and between each other. Principles continually serve as a template for team members to use to assess whether the foundations and expectations of team performance and behavior are being continually fulfilled as the team goes about its usual and routine activities.

NEW RULES FOR THE ORGANIZATION

To create the integrated, whole systems, team-driven organization that results in a streamlined, efficient, and competitive environment, a continuing commitment to innovation, creativity, and point-of-service must be present. The structure must support the change effort and help facilitate the building of a team-based approach and a continuum of service. Leadership in the health system must create a true point-of-service continuum of care that effectively addresses the continuing health of those who comprise the system's subscriber population.

This indicates a need to create an organization committed to learning, unfolding, creativity, and change. Some conditions are defined that require a tightening of the organization's parameters in efficiency and effectiveness in both design and process. Some initial activities are necessary to ensure the appropriate configuration of the organization in support of its team-based and effective delineation.

1. **No more job orientation**. All work in a system is specifically directed to the outcomes of the organization. The organization must be lean and effective in a way that better meets the needs of those the organization serves and better exemplifies the role and relationship of the providers. An organization should be made up of highly trained, efficient, and effective workers supported by associates who can help provide functional support to the work. Team-based activities will demand a tight fit between the kind, number, and quality of workers and the expectations to which their work is directed.

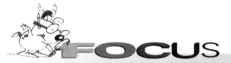

FOCUS

Innovation requires a commitment to experimentation. Everyone should feel safe to experiment and fail. Error and failure are essential to any success. Indeed, there is no success without error. Therefore error should be:

- A cause for celebration
- An element of measurement
- A signpost of progress
- A pause for study
- A foundation for correction
- Anticipated before it occurs
- A safe moment for evaluation

It is the end of the "job" age. As the Industrial Age passes, those elements that reflect it also pass. In the new world of work, roles are more mobile, fluid, and flexible, reflecting a wide variety of content. Behaviors now must reflect these new conditions or suffer the loss of new opportunities.

There is an inverse relationship between the number of managers and an efficient organization. The more managers an organization has, the more managers it needs. In truth, any system should have only enough managers to support its work and not a person more!

Information is the life's blood of any system. Increasing commitment to building good information systems is essential to future success. The more a system is driven from its point-of-service, the more information it needs to have available to the decision makers there.

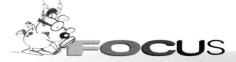

Function is no longer the foundation for effectiveness in service provision; fit is. In systems, the fit between process and outcome, structure and work, mission and service, and consumer and provider is the measure of a strong organization. Fit requires:

• A commitment to building good relationships between providers
• Customer-oriented service providers
• Clear understanding of the work
• Orientation to achieving outcomes
• Good knowledge of integration and systems processes
• Sound evaluation process

2. **The organization should have as little management structure as possible.** In team-based designs, the intent of the system is to create effective decision making at the point-of-service. The providers and partners should be not only capable but willing to make effective decisions where service is provided. In addition, the system must be configured to support that point-of-service decision making. This requires as few managers as possible in the system, only enough to maintain the integrity of the system. As the continuum becomes more clearly developed the point-of-service becomes better defined, and the need for **management-controlled** decisions diminishes. The decision-making expertise, incorporation of meaningful information, and **evaluation of the** effectiveness of work more often will occur among the team members at the point-of-service.

3. **Use of data to drive decision making is increasing.** The architecture of the future of all health care systems is the information infrastructure. Information is a river that flows through any system. Any member of a system and any team that does the work of the system should be able to "dip" into the river of information and obtain from it whatever information is needed to support the work and effective decision making of that team or member. Both the knowledgeable worker and the information infrastructure are increasingly the key capital of future health care organizations. The tightness of fit between the ability of the knowledgeable worker to achieve outcomes and the information that supports process and evaluation are critical to effectiveness, quality, and service sustainability.

4. **Build a tightness of fit between what the organization provides and what the consumer needs.** In the past providers in health care structures determined what consumers needed and generated those services within the constructs providers created. In a health-driven service system the partnership between providers and consumers is essential to determine the character and content of appropriate ser-

vices on the part of the system. Therefore a stronger intersection and communication is required between provider and subscriber in the health care system. Increasingly, the system is obliged to keep the subscriber healthy in order to reduce cost and achieve a level of continuing health status. To do that, commitment, investment, and involvement on the part of both provider and consumer in an equity-based relationship must exist. Therefore the system increasingly must be sensitive to how well its services are integrated with the demand for those services that come out of its subscriber relationship. This fit between service and need is critical to service effectiveness and systems viability.

Although certainly not comprehensive, each of these items has a critical impact on the effectiveness of team-based approaches to service delivery. The ability to continue and maintain team-based approaches depends predominantly on how many of these processes are attended to within the organizational system. The leader must recognize that moving to team-based approaches means more than simply the creation of teams and the facilitation of their development. It requires a structural shift, a thinking shift, involving major adjustments in both the construction and operation of the organizational system.

From every level of leadership through every point-of-service the organization must reflect a different framework for service and must be driven by a different set of variables, moving from the point-of-service throughout the supporting organizational system, into its operational and administrative structures, and out through its board and back through its community. And the reverse must operate as fluidly and as effectively from the community through its board, administrative, operational, and service structures back to the point-of-service where the community is served, one member at a time. This seamless, fluid flow of decision making must be supported by a system whose purpose it is to maintain the fluidity, flexibility, and integration of the system around the continuum of relationships that comprise it.

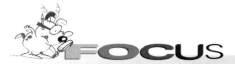

Creating a team-based organization is more than simply constructing teams. It means changing the thinking of the organization and seeing with different eyes:
- Horizontal rather than hierarchical relationships
- Collective outcomes rather than individual functions
- Evaluating outcomes and not simply processes
- Focusing on the point-of-service
- Creating a tightness of fit between consumer and provider

Seamlessness is the creation of good interfaces between each component of the system: governance, operations, and service. It recognizes that each component must support the other to create an effective and lasting system.

THE SYSTEM AS NETWORK

As discussed earlier, the old hierarchical, vertically designed structures are outmoded. Thus far we have outlined many of the reasons for this. The question remains, what models are emerging for organizational systems that support team-based activities?

Increasingly, on the health care horizon, newer designs for organization that are more horizontally oriented and continuum based are emerging as the predominant framework for the structuring of health care services. Because it is increasingly important to link services together in a comprehensive array of programs to meet managed care and consumer demands, health care services are changing their designs to support service integration across the system. The needs of a service-integrated organization across a continuum of service structures requires a different format than institutionally based, functionally focused service structures (Box 2-3).

As these new horizontal patterns of organizational configuration emerge, new kinds of relationships also are engendered. These relationships reflect a more equity-based foundation and require a higher level of dialogue, problem solving, service integration, and relationship building across the system. Furthermore, they require a network of intersections both within the support structures and the service framework of the organization. All of this serves as the foundation for the formation of a more networked orientation to the design of organizations.

Networks are a web of intersecting and interrelating functions and relationships that contain an array of connections exemplifying the set of relationships necessary to the integrity and service of a system. Networks are relationship intensive. As a result, they require a high level of interaction, communication, and information. In fact, networks are information dependent. A successful network requires an information infrastructure that continually flows through the system and permits its members to have access to whatever information resources they need to make good decisions, render good judgments, and evaluate the effectiveness of their relationship and their work together. At every level of a network system, people need

Health Care Service Integration

Newer models of organizations are emerging that exemplify the movement toward systems design. In health care they personify the following:
1. Integration
2. Linkage
3. Continuum
4. Teams
5. Partnership
6. Clinical pathways
7. Strong service orientation

Health systems increasingly look like webs rather than pyramids. The reality of necessary intersecting structures and relationships is changing the shape and design of structures supporting a continuum of health care services.

to directly access the resources and information necessary to function appropriately, as well as produce and evaluate outcomes (Team Tip 2-2).

In a clinical organization, such as a health care system, generation of information and development of communication networks are critical to the work of health service delivery. There is no room for error in the communication of information about patients, their conditions, and their needs in evaluating the effects of intervention. In a network system this need is extended by the fact that decisions are made across the system and depend on other decisions made at other points in the information and communication network.

In a fundamental way teams are networks, too. Just as individuals on teams depend on the fluidity and fit of other individuals on the team, systems depend on the fit of teams with each other. A network can be visualized as an array of concentric circles crossing each other, cross-referenced and related, tied together by common purposes, and linked by the information and communication channels necessary to sustain them.

Just as networks are necessary to build the structure that defines the relationship between service providers and service structures, support systems also are required (Box 2-4). An intersecting and interacting array of support processes to those who provide service is necessary to ensure that the resources needed to continue services are available in the manner required. In a network system, support services form the outer boundaries, whereas the supporting periphery is located around point-of-service systems to continually support, supply, and evaluate the distribution and use of resources across the system. Every service team needs to have the confidence that what is required to perform the work will be available in a way that is facilitating and time sensitive. In most organizations, a predominating concern for the point-of-service worker is not so much whether he or she achieves a quality of service, but rather whether the system supports consistently are in place so that essential resources are available.

The foundation for success and sustainability is created by the successful continuous integration of organizational, support, and service networks

TEAM**TIP**   2.2

Readily Available Resources

The health professional must be able to render good judgement about the patient he or she serves. That means having necessary information readily available in a form that can be understood and useful. They should not need to struggle with the system to get the basic support needed to provide good service. They need:
1. *Simple documentation.*
2. *Easy access.*
3. *Patient-specific data.*
4. *Direct communication*
5. *Immediate feedback.*

BOX **2-4**

Networks and Support Systems

Networks and support systems work hand in hand to ensure that people have what is necessary to do their work. This partnership between the network and its supports must:
- Ensure easy access to information
- Provide supplies and equipment on demand
- Provide costs as they are accrued
- Validate the clinical choices of the provider
- Ensure quick evaluation data of the fit between needs and choices
- Assist the provider in any corrective actions needed

Newer models of organization, such as shared governance, create the structure that represents focus on systems, integration, continuum, and point-of-service, as well as the empowered, linked processes necessary to support service in integrated health systems.

in the system. Each of the components of the organization must intersect with the other in a seamless way that ensures all elements of the system converge around the purposes and services it provides. This increasingly is important in a decentralized, horizontally configured, continuum-based health care system. The linkages across the system become vital to the ability of the system to make decisions in a decentralized way and provide the services in the varied places where it will emerge in a managed care, capitated health care delivery system.

Newer models of system design, such as shared governance, shared leadership, whole systems management, systems teams, empowerment, and a range of associated structural designs, are signs of experimentation to support the point-of-service and the decision making necessary there. Each of these structural approaches and models must be modified to support the culture within which they unfold. Clearly, in a multifocal health care delivery system, no one approach is appropriate for all settings.

The principles that support models and approaches must be consistent across the system. If the principles of partnership, equity, accountability, and ownership are the themes running through the design of any struc-

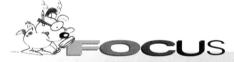

The seamless connections among components of the organization ensure all members that:
1. A real system exists for support of their work.
2. Each component of the organization is supporting other processes to which they relate.
3. All the pieces of the system are coming together to support its work.
4. Linkage between each related element of the system is tight and facilitates relationships.
5. Providers can get the necessary tools to do their work and feel the support of the system for them.

tural or model approach to building support, team-based organizations, those structures remain viable. If the principles are inconsistent, are controlling, provide inadequate support, shift the locus of control from where it belongs, or reintroduce a high level of hierarchy, they begin to diminish the effectiveness of team-based approaches. A consonance between the structural models, operational decision-making processes, and organizational structure must be present if team-based activities and decision making are to be consistently supported and reinforced. The consonance between structure, process, and outcome remains a centerpiece to the effectiveness of design and the workings of a team-based organizational system.

CHANGING THE SERVICE SYSTEM

The initiation of horizontally configured and continuum-based structures changes the entire character of the institution and service environment. Processes associated with managing and leading the continuum are not what they were in past institutional models, which were isolated and compartmentalized on illness-based interventions. While the good portion of illness care services will continue to be offered within institutions (after all, people will continue to become sick), the broad goal of the health care system and its services is to reduce the need for high-intensity, sickness-based services among its subscribers to the fullest extent possible (Box 2-5). This attempt to achieve the goal of health in the system creates an entirely different dynamic in the structure, delivery, and management of health services.

In team-based approaches the partnerships embedded in the teams require deliberation and decision making among the team's members. Indeed, up to 90% of decisions that affect provider-patient interaction will be made at the point-of-service. To ensure that this happens at a high level of effectiveness and efficiency, the leadership and support roles of the system must be such that it is possible for team members to be successful in decision making and to have the skills and freedom necessary to voice these decisions. Teams should be essentially self-managed and self-directed. Although team members are highly interdependent, interaction depends on both facilitating leadership and team skill development.

BOX 2-5

Health Care of the Future

Much of health care in the future will be provided outside the hospital. As health systems build a strong continuum of services, the locus of control in the system shifts from the institution to the service. Wherever service is provided it is also controlled. Two things will be required:

1. Information infrastructure at the point-of-service where it is portable, comprehensive, and immediate
2. Competent, well prepared providers who can act interdependently with other providers and independently from the hospital.

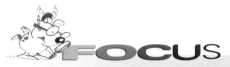

Teams naturally function interdependently. Still, teamwork has not been a "normal" mode of function in health care. While providers have access to each other and cross one another's paths frequently, they can do so and still not have a relationship. Teams are built on relationships. Therefore:

- Physicians will have to learn new behaviors to be effective in teams in the future.
- A stronger relationship between provider roles will need to be clarified.
- Time together must be defined for doing the work of team building.
- Building critical service pathways will require a clarification of every team member's role.

The clinical staff has the obligation for building effective teams. Team building should not be driven from "above" in the system or there would be no ownership from those who make the team thrive. The structure should remove everything in the system that prevents teams from becoming the modus operandi for the way service is provided.

The movement from manager to leader is a critical one and a challenging journey. Much of the expectations of the manager role, in terms of planning, organizing, leading, controlling, and directing, is no longer an appropriate framework for the activities of leadership. Because teams need to operate interdependently; make effective decisions; and have the skills necessary to deliberate, make judgments, problem solve, solution seek, and assess quality, much of the role of leader focuses on facilitating those activities rather than undertaking those activities herself. Old management behaviors are not suitable for this environment. The leadership behaviors that are appropriate require a different set of processes, some of which will necessitate education on the part of the manager becoming leader.

The organization and system that support team-based activities cannot continue to act as parent or in a supervisor-subordinate manner. Administrative and management goals and desires, like those of members of the teams, must be subject to discernment, exploration, and validation. The dialogue across the system necessary to determine the viability of those supports involves all of the stakeholders, whether they be managers or staff team members. The staff members who comprise the teams should not have to accept demands, rules, notions, or plans that affect what they do without their participation and evaluation of the appropriateness in facilitating their work. Therefore vertical models of position and control have less value in a system than do the abilities to integrate, facilitate, and coordinate decision making in relationship building across the system in support of team activities. In organizations using systems models that support team-based activities, action undertaken in one part of the system affects activities and functions throughout the system. These implications are apparent to all who make up the service base of the organization. Relationship, not control, is essential to the integrity of team-based approaches and the effectiveness of the system.

Continuum-based approaches to designing the organization, team-based decision making, and functional processes require a significant change in management, administrative work, and support in the organization. The way in which management and leadership work with each other requires changing the pattern of the organizational system. These newer expectations emerge in a way that demands a significant shift in the role of every health care leader in a team-based approach. Some shifting expectations include the following:

1. Decisions about the supporting mission, purpose, and objectives are made in the context of the whole system, thus including all the partners who make up the system's team-based activities.

2. From the board of trustees through the functional teams, all members of the system are partners in decision-making processes. Each one has the task of ensuring that appropriate linkages exist between all components of the system, both operational and service, and create a tight fit to the community they serve.

3. Horizontal integration requires that vertical systems support relationships across the continuum. Relationships are critical to the viability of health care decision making. Building relationships between teams and across the system is the major work of leadership.

4. Teams do not compete with each other. If any competition does exist, it is within the team and its relationship to its own goals, expectations, and performance standards. The role of leadership is to constantly facilitate the improvement of team performance to ensure that the services provided are of the highest quality and produce the best outcomes. If a team succeeds in evidencing high levels of excellence, it need never worry about competing with other teams.

5. Partnering is critical, ongoing work in any team-based organization. The quality of partnering along the continuum of care is central to the success of the organization. Leadership's role is to support, facilitate, problem solve, and create learning opportunities for the enrichment and expansion of partnering behaviors at the team level and throughout the system.

6. The primary role of a leader is to nurture the relationships in the system. Continuum of care systems are built on strong, mutually

All systems need a process that interfaces the strategy established at the governance level with the tactics that come from the operations leadership of the system and with the service objectives that come from the providers who do the work of the health system.

41

defined relationships and interactions. Leadership offers the kind of support and guidance that strengthens relationships, builds skills in maintaining them, and helps in problem solving when relationships are challenged or broken.

7. Much of the role of leadership relates to the creation and mainte-nance of linkages throughout the system. At the administrative, op-erations, and service levels of the system, seamless intersections, support connections, relationship linkages, problem solving, and solution seeking throughout the system are critical elements of the leader's role. At every level and place in the system where leader-ship exists, the focus is to facilitate the effectiveness of team-based function and the relationship of teams to those they serve and to each other.

8. Team-based approaches to work and decision making do not re-quire intervention and control from the management structure of the system. The need for intervention represents a failure of leader-ship (Team Tip 2-3). Teams are self-managed processes. They re-quire continual resources, support, information, tools, and develop-ment. These elements are the focus of the leader. If resources and support are present and appropriate, leadership will never need to worry about the character and quality of the work produced by the system.

9. Public evaluation of the performance of the system and its teams is a must in consumer-driven organizations. Patient care requires that systems determine the effectiveness of its processes, structures, and supports, as evidenced by the satisfaction, quality, efficacy, and effec-tiveness of strategies along the continuum of care. Evaluation of per-formance and outcomes provides all members of a system, those who provide service and those who are served, with the essential informa-tion about the efficacy and viability of the service structure in place.

Clearly, leadership roles require a different set of behaviors and expecta-tions. In team-based approaches the leader is viewed as partner, facilitator,

---

TEAM**TIP**   2.3

Self-management

Managers should never control clinical teams. The purpose of the team is to make decisions about the accountability that reflects the team's work. The manager is obligated to ensure that skills resulting in good decisions, rela-tionships, and service are present in all team members. Beyond that, the manager should have no func-tional or decision-making role with the team. The mature and functioning team is always self-directed.

coach, teacher, and role model. These behaviors require a sense of related-ness, value, and partnership with all the players of the team. The consistent unfolding of the leader's role, and its application across the system, will strengthen leadership and provide the kinds of resources and support that teams need to thrive and achieve their intended outcomes.

STRUCTURING FOR CONSENSUS

Team-based approaches require entirely different processes from those of past hierarchical management structures. Team-driven organizational systems require different methods to achieve outcomes and undertake the processes that support those outcomes. New models of interaction and decision making must emerge at the heart of the system if it is to operate effectively in team-based approaches.

Consensus decision-making models are the preferred framework for effective decision making within the organizational system (Box 2-6). Consensus is not agreement. Consensus is not voting in support of decision making. Instead, it is the convergence of all process and relationships around activities that reflect what is right for the organization and the people who comprise it. Consensus represents a level of understanding on the part of all participants that the right decision must be achieved and, therefore, arrived at through defined, disciplined processes among the members of the organization.

In a team-driven organization the use of time and relationship is essential to the quality of decision making. Therefore the judicious and appropriate use of time is critical to the effectiveness of decision making in team-based systems.

Discipline, dialogue, and interaction are critical to the effectiveness of decision making in team-based approaches. Teams must use method and technique in effective dialogue and decision-making processes. The use of Continuous Quality Improvement (CQI) techniques for assessing process; the use of consensus-building approaches to the deliberation of problems; and the need for resolution, utilizing tools for problem solving, and

BOX **2-6**

Consensus Models with the Organization

Consensus models of problem solving and decision making are the method of preference for team-based organizations. Consensus requires that the organization be willing to:
- Allow team members to solve their own problems
- Have specific performance goals around which the team can configure its work
- Develop a consistent method for team problem solving and deliberation that can be replicated
- Initiate a learning process for teams in need of skill building in team dynamics

Consensus is not agreement. It is a process for working through a diversity of contributions with methods that help the participants find common ground from which they can build relationship and response.

process-oriented mechanisms for deliberation, as well as quality activities in measurement devices, all are requisites of team-based interaction in dynamics. CQI is not a structure or system. Instead, it is a set of methods and processes that improve action and work to ensure a strong fit between methods and outcomes. The elements of CQI will shift as demand and focus are altered. CQI supports systems models of service, it does not define them. The idea of disciplining dialogue, process, and relationship is critical to effectiveness. Work teams are not social bodies; their meaning and purpose is directly related to the work around which they configure. Therefore the issues regarding work drives the content of their dialogue and relationship. Teams must focus on activities that relate to who they are and what they do. The development of systems and techniques, tools, and resources that facilitate effective dialogue and decision making are essential to the efficiency and effectiveness of team-based decision making, processing, and evaluating.

Much of the activity of team relationship and intersection is reflected in how much the team deals with the behaviors and interaction among its members. A shift to team-based dynamics will create major behavioral changes, requiring much discussion and interaction as people adjust to new ways of relating and behaving. This interaction must be accommodated, and method and technique must be applied to ensure that the dialogue is focused and results in meaningful behavioral changes. Much of this book is devoted to the methods and techniques needed to facilitate the functions and activities of teams.

Significant structural changes in the organization must occur to support the behavioral and relationship shifts to team-based organizational and decision-making systems. Major commitments on the part of every member of the system, from board of trustees through point-of-service, are required. Each component of the organization must assess itself and raise questions about how it supports the development of functional and effective decision making that influences the quality of service in the places where health care is provided. Across the system, each partner and member of the organization has an obligation to create the circumstances and conditions that lead to successful interaction and relationship at the team level (Team Tip 2-4). This requires new structures as well as new insights and behaviors. Each of these must link in a way that creates the environment and circumstances necessary to support the outcomes of team-based activities. Without the convergence of each of these new structures around the relationships of team members at the point-of-service, the relationships between and among teams and the outcomes of their work will be measurably constrained. When these components converge to support the activities of the team, they facilitate not only relationships but also achievement of high quality and meaningful outcomes in the relationships among team members and between the team-based system and those it serves. After all, meeting patients' needs is the purpose of any health care organization.

> ### TEAM**TIP**   2.4
> *Partners Across the System*
> All partners in a system are members of that system and have rights and obligations to the system and to each other. These rights and obligations must be clearly defined by the members, providing a baseline from which team members can evaluate the team and each other. This establishes the foundation for individual commitment and for group relationships.

Bibliography

Ackoff R: *The democratic corporation,* New York, Oxford University Press, 1994.

Alexander J, Zuckerman H, Pointer D: The challenges of governing integrated health systems, *Health Care Management Review* 20(4):69-81, 1995.

Ashkenas R et al: *The boundaryless organization,* San Francisco, Jossey-Bass, 1995.

Aubry R, Cohen P: *Working wisdom,* San Francisco, Jossey-Bass, 1995.

Beckham D: Ownership—the longest lever, *Healthcare Forum Journal,* 39(1):48-54, 1996.

Beckhard R, Pritchard W: *Changing the essence: the art of creating and leading fundamental change in organizations,* San Francisco, Jossey-Bass, 1992.

Belasco J, Gorham G: Why empowerment does not empower: the bankruptcy of current paradigms, *Seminars for Nurse Managers* 4(1):20-27, 1996.

Beneveniste G: *The twenty-first century organization,* San Francisco, Jossey-Bass, 1994.

Bennis W, Biederman P: *Organizing genius,* New York, Addison-Wesley, 1997.

Bolman L, Terrance D: *Reframing organizations,* San Francisco, Jossey-Bass, 1997.

Chawla S, Renesch J: *Learning organizations: developing cultures for tomorrows workplace,* Portland, Or, Productivity Press, 1995.

Cox Jr T: *Cultural diversity in organizations,* San Francisco, Berrett-Koehler, 1993.

Drucker P: The new society of organizations, Sept/Oct: 95-104, 1992.

Evans K et al: Whole systems shared governance: a model for the integrated health system, *Journal of Nursing Administration* 25(5):18-27, 1995.

Galbraith J: *Designing organizations,* San Francisco, Jossey-Bass, 1995.

Gould J, DiBella A, Nevis E: Organizations as learning systems, *The Systems Thinker* 4(8):1-3, 1993.

Halal W: *The new management: democracy and enterprise,* San Francisco, Berrett-Koehler, 1996.

Handy C: *Beyond certainty: the changing world of organizations,* Boston, Harvard Business School Press, 1996.

Harman W, Porter M: *The new business of business,* San Francisco, Berrett-Koehler, 1997.

Harrison B: *Lean and mean: the changing landscape of corporate power in the age of flexibility,* New York, Basic Books, 1994.

Hock D: The chaordic organization: out of chaos into order, *World Business Academy Perspectives* 9(1):5-18, 1995.

Hurst D: *Crisis & renewal,* Boston, Harvard Business School Press, 1995.

Jamieson D, O'Mara J: *Managing workforce 2000,* San Francisco, Jossey-Bass, 1991.

Janov J: *The inventive organization: hope and daring at work,* San Francisco, Jossey-Bass, 1994.

Keidel R: *Seeing organizational patterns,* San Francisco, Berrett-Koehler, 1995.

Kets de Vries M, Miller D: *The neurotic organization,* San Francisco, Jossey-Bass, 1984.

Kim D: *Toward learning organizations,* Cambridge, Mass, Pegasus Communication, 1992.

Korten D: *When corporations rule the world,* San Francisco, Berrett-Koehler, 1995.

Lawler, E, Mohrman S, Ledford G: *Creating high performance organizations,* San Francisco, Jossey-Bass, 1995.

Lawler III E: *Motivation in work organizations,* San Francisco, Jossey-Bass, 1994.

Luthans F, Hodgetts R, Lee S: New paradigm organizations, *Organizational Dynamics* 22(3):5-19, 1994.

Marszalek-Gaucher E, Coffey R: *Transforming healthcare organizations: how to achieve and sustain organizational excellence,* San Francisco, Jossey-Bass, 1990.

Merry M: Shared leadership in healthcare organizations, *Topics in Health Care Financing* 20(4):26-38, 1994.

Mink O et al: *Open organizations,* San Francisco, Jossey-Bass, 1994.

Mohrman S, Cohen S, Mohrman A: *Designing team based organizations,* San Francisco, Jossey-Bass, 1995.

Mohrman S, Mohrman A: *Designing and leading team based organizations,* San Francisco, Jossey-Bass, 1997.

Nielson D: Partnering with employees, San Francisco, Jossey-Bass, 1993.

Nirenberg J: *The living organization: transforming teams into workplace communities,* Homewood, Ill, Irwin Professional Publishing, 1993.

Nolan R, Croson D: *Creative destruction: a six stage process for transforming organizations,* Boston, Harvard Business School Press, 1995.

Oshry B: *Seeing systems, unlocking the mysteries of organizational life,* San Francisco, Berrett-Koehler, 1995.

Pauchant T, Mitroft I: *Transforming the crisis prone organization,* San Francisco, Jossey-Bass, 1992.

Pedersen A, Easton L: Teamwork: bringing order out of chaos, *Nursing Management* 26(6):34-35, 1995.

Poirier C, Reiter S: *Supply chain optimization,* San Francisco, Berrett-Koehler, 1996.

Schein E: On dialogue, culture, and organizational learning, {AU: JOURNAL TITLE??} 22(2):40-51, 1993.

Shortell S et al: The holographic organization, 36(2):20-25, 1993.

Treece J: Breaking the chains of command: when information technology alters the workplace, *Business Week* p. 112-114, 1994.

Vogt J, Murrell K: *Empowerment in organizations,* San Diego, Calif, University Associates, Inc, 1990.

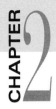

TOOLCHEST

TOOL A: Checklist for Integration

Health care organizations are in the midst of developing integrated team-based approaches across the continuum of care. All transformation and integration related to integration depends on:

1. The strategies that are undertaken to respond to the demand for change
2. The unique culture and characteristics of the organization as it addresses this change
3. The willingness and ability of the organization to undertake its necessary activities in order to adjust and adapt to its dynamic changing circumstances

INTEGRATION CHECKLIST

Instructions. Each of the following items should be identified and checked off as part of successful integration processes. It is critical that each element in integrating team-based approaches be in place and support the team-based activities.

1. Identification of the environmental and market forces that create the conditions for change and the necessary response to them.

Initiation of horizontal collaborative systems rather than institutional competition.

Reduction in all high-end cost and excess capacity, impeding the organization's responsiveness to change.

Tightening of the framework of workers and creation of a closer alignment of the number of workers with the leanness of the organization.

Provision of broad-based, comprehensive range of service, facilitating access between payers, providers, and consumers.

Reduction of cost in as many places as possible.

Advanced pricing formulas, first introduced through discounting processes and later unfolding as advanced and fixed pricing mechanisms for the organization.

Sufficient availability of capital for investing in horizontally aligned health care service across the continuum of care.

2. Response to individual systems' culture and environment.

The system builds on the mission, purposes, and objectives of its community responsibility for providing health care for a defined population over a range of services.

Each participant has a defined role and accountability in the system, including group, organization, and individual provider participants.

An organizational model and framework for integrated delivery of care is point-of-service-driven, team-based, and integrated across the continuum of service.

A planned, carefully constructed transition from the old health care system to a new model of integration is defined and outlined.

There are clearly delineated clinical pathways, or centers of excellence, where specific population-based services are provided.

There is clear linkage between all systems services and support services driven by a strongly developed information infrastructure.

Management structures are diminished, limited, and efficiently defined, so that there are as few managers as the system requires.

The system represents a full range of comprehensive services to the community or population it serves and becomes a one-stop health care system for its consumers.

Team-based approaches, standards, and decision making are facilitated across the system in effective clinical models representing clear delineation of points of service.

Physicians are involved in every phase of the clinical process and development and are incorporated in all decisions that affect the design and service structure of the system.

3. A new organization emerges with a new organizational culture and mindset.

The change is difficult, requiring time, patience, and consistency. Leadership expresses this.

Team-based approaches align and create incentives for team members to fully participate and express ownership in the change.

All integration is relationship-building. The organization, increasingly, is a horizontal, relationship-driven entity.

Structuring based on the value of relationships is critical to the success of the system.

Systems approaches require a view of the whole rather than of the parts.

Comprehensive integrated, aligned arrangement of services and structures should reflect the whole commitment of the organization's specific service to its community.

Integration is a journey, not an event. It continues to adjust, change, modify, moderate, and advance as each stage unfolds.

Each of the elements are critical to effective change in the organizational system and must be addressed as part of building the team-based approach.

TOOL B: Confronting the Team-Building Myths

In *Team Building for the Future*, R.L. Elledge and S.L. Phillips* identify 20 myths of team building. Each of these myths represents a particular set of

behaviors that build on the myths. This exercise takes those 20 myths and asks questions about their legitimacy in the team-building process in any organization. Building team process on truth, frank-

*Elledge RL, Phillips SL: *Team building for the future*, San Diego, Pfeiffer & Co, 1994.

ness, and clarity is an important construct for sustainable teams. Making sure that myth is not present is critical to the effectiveness of team process.

Myth No. 1

Facilitators are objective third-party consultants.
How do you generate this myth in your organization?
Do you support the facilitator as a human being?
Do you allow for growth and development of the facilitator?
Is the facilitator vulnerable and open to growth and change?

Myth No. 2

Facilitators will transfer their team-building skills to the team.
Does the facilitator have sufficient skill to transfer?
Is the facilitator confident of his or her skills?
Are the processes of skill transfer in place within the team?
Does the team trust the facilitator enough to look to her or him for skill transfer?
Is a format available for the transfer of skills to team members?

Myth No. 3

Teams develop in a steady, predictable series of phases.
Do the issues of growth get reflected in the concerns that the team raises?
Is the team allowed to revisit issues when it continues to have problems?
Is the team's developmental cycle evaluated for the effectiveness of team members and their learning?

Is learning a dynamic process depending on the needs of the team and the timing of those needs?
Does the team change its structure and format if they no longer fits its needs?
If interaction is a problem, can the team change its process and format to facilitate it better?
Is the team allowed to go back and forth as needed to address what it does well and the developments that it has yet to address?
Can the team evaluate its effectiveness and adjust its processes according to its results?
Can the team accommodate the growth needs of an individual member, allowing time for change to occur but requiring change nonetheless?
Does the team realize that change is highly adjustable and cyclical?
Is the team willing to do remedial work and address concerns that affect advanced work on the team?

Myth No. 4

All effective leaders undertake team building.
Do leaders understand the team-building process?
Does the leader monitor and adjust his or her skill based on the team's development?
Has the team leader participated in planning for activities related to team building?
Has the team leader identified specific skills he or she needs in the team-building process?

Myth No. 5

All team members are equal in team-building interventions.
Does the leader include all team members in dialogue?

Have all team members participated in identifying their team's learning objectives?

Are the roles of team members clear enough for members to know what development they must undertake?

Will the team be willing to engage team building as an endless, timeless process?

Is the team willing to clarify and communicate the issues of concern as they arise, realizing they may set the team back developmentally?

Can the team deal with a sometimes schizophrenic roller-coaster ride between effectiveness and developmental needs?

Can the team adjust to the changing work requirements and the environmental changes that either impede or facilitate team process?

Can the team live with the continuously dynamic, ever growing need to adjust skills, change behaviors, and advance the process of the team?

Myth No. 6

Teams change, adjust, and improve their operations and then restabilize.

Is it understood that the team moves incrementally and noncharacteristically between all stages of development?

Is there a model for change that the team uses to validate its shifts and growth?

Can the team live with the chaos and complexity associated with change?

Myth No. 7

In team building, consensus decision making is always best.

Is there a consensus process within the team?

Does the team know how to use the consensus process?

Is there a method for conflict resolution?

Is solution seeking the framework for team process?

Is there method and technique applied to consensus building in the team?

Myth No. 8

Teams can perceive, analyze, and decide in a logical deductive manner.

Are there a method and framework for problem solving in the team?

Are the problem activities of the team associated with its plan?

Are the individual objectives of members consistent with those of the team?

Do the team's process and outcomes fit with the purposes and goals of the system?

Is there accommodation for the adjustments and changes that invariably occur in any system?

Myth No. 9

An objective reality exists that can be understood.

Is there a clear understanding that reality is not a straight line?

Do people look at the whole rather than simply the parts?

Can team members read the signposts of change rather than focus only on the end point?

Does the team honor a variety of perceptions, including subjective and changing perceptions?

Myth No. 10

The factors that influence our perceptions are fully known.

Is there respect given to the growth that comes from discovery?

Is it safe on the team to ask for clarification?

Do team members clearly understand the meaning of the issues under discussion?

Is there generalized agreement on the awareness of the team around the issues of discussion?

Is there a way to build perception more strongly as the team seeks consensus?

Myth No. 11

All team members must be fully committed to the team's vision and goals.

Is there room for diversity and a variety of perceptions around how the team achieves its goals?

Is there commitment to determination of common efforts around goals?

Can the team allow a minority of perceptions that do not generally agree with those of the majority of team members?

Does the team have a way of getting clear ideas of those different perceptions that contribute to good dialogue?

Is diversity on the team expected and honored?

Myth No. 12

One person's performance can be looked at independently of another's.

Is there realization that team members are interdependent?

Can team members honor the perceptions of others in a way that incorporates it into the work, solution seeking, planning, or problem solving?

Do individual members see themselves as part of the team?

Does a feedback mechanism exist to support the contributions of team members?

Can the separateness of individuals coalesce around a common set of goals?

Myth No. 13

Synergy is the end result of team work.

Is there room for the growth of cooperation and inspiration?

Is there an understanding that each individual makes a contribution to the whole?

Is it clear what the expectations for performance are for each individual?

Does the team accommodate the development of individuals toward its goals and outcomes?

Myth No. 14

A team-building facilitator enables a team to learn about itself.

Is there room for "what if" scenarios in the learning process?

Does the team facilitator have a variety of techniques that help the team past its barriers?

Does the team respect the facilitator's work?

Does the facilitator incorporate the notions of diversity of perception and role into problem solving?

Does the facilitation result in advancing the team's skill set and independence in making its own decisions?

Myth No. 15

A team-building intervention is controlled by the team's leader.

Does leadership always rest in the hands of the team facilitator or coordinator?

Is leadership allowed to emerge as needed within specific processes of the team's work?

The data collected from a team are always confidential and anonymous.

Is it clear which data are confidential and which data are not?

Should all data be anonymous, or can it be determined which are and which are not?

Can work process and data related to it ever be fully confidential?

How open should sessions be; how closed should they be?

When confidential information is shared is there a mechanism for ensuring it remains confidential?

Myth No. 16

Interventions are designed to fit the needs of the team.

Is the team clear about what interventions or actions result in meaningful outcomes?

Is there a variety of styles that fit the needs of the team regarding its leadership?

Does the facilitator exhibit skill in confronting issues?

Can the facilitator demonstrate empathy?

Is the facilitator good at encouraging the team in analyzing its own processes?

Is the facilitator articulate?

Myth No. 17

Trust is dependent on complete openness and candor.

Does the team understand that trust is the result of good team dynamics, not its cause?

Can trust be enumerated once the team focuses on identifying it?

Does the team trust that diversity will lead to appropriate integration and meaningful outcomes?

Is the team clear about its expectations and relationships?

Is there an individual team member development plan that can be used to evaluate effective team building?

Is there discipline that allows for intervention when team building indicates a problem?

Myth No. 18

Facilitators work with a variety of options for team structures and interactions.

Does the team know the level of creativity and innovation used in facilitating its process?

Does the team reflect a tightness of fit between its design and the culture it serves?

Is the team fluid and flexible in design in the application of its work?

Does the team assess the effectiveness of its facilitation and the congruence with its outcomes and work?

Myth No. 19

Is leadership facilitated by the coordinator and facilitator of the team?

Does the team's leadership change periodically in order to create a dynamic growth of leadership on the team?

Can the facilitator encourage the emergence of leadership in others as a part of his or her work?

Myth No. 20

Team building is a continuous process.

Does the team realize that team building is a dynamic?

Does the team have a measure of its successes?

Does the team know how to deal directly with its failures?

Each of these myths raises questions about the team's own reality and its possibility for success. Team development must continually address its interactions, behaviors, formats, and functions.

TOOL C: Shared Governance Staff Assessment Instrument

Instructions: This instrument provides you with the opportunity to assess your work roles and behaviors within the context of a shared governance organizational framework. This assessment provides you with an opportunity to determine the impact of shared governance on your work and role.

To use this instrument read the statements carefully. Choose your answer after consideration by selecting the response that best matches your personal feelings and the extent to which you agree with the statements below. Mark the corresponding space on your response sheet. Please complete all the statements and remember, you cannot be identified, so be frank in selecting the response that matches as closely as possible to your own view.

Part A: Survey

	1	2	3	4	5
1. Shared governance is a system of management that allows staff participation.	1	2	3	4	5
2. Shared governance changes the way we relate to each other.	1	2	3	4	5
3. In shared governance, staff members make more decisions.	1	2	3	4	5
4. Our organization sincerely wants shared governance to work	1	2	3	4	5
5. Staff will never let shared governance work here.	1	2	3	4	5
6. I believe in shared governance.	1	2	3	4	5
7. Shared governance is the key element in what keeps me working here.	1	2	3	4	5
8. Shared governance is just a fad that won't last long.	1	2	3	4	5
9. The processes associated with shared governance are consistent with my manager's style of management.	1	2	3	4	5

Part B: Attitudes

On a scale of 1 to 10, with 1 the lowest and 10 the highest, please rank the following:

1. I believe the overall commitment to shared governance in this organization ranks _____.

2. I believe the quality of interpersonal relationships in this organization rank   _____.

3. I believe the overall leadership ability in this organization rank   _____.

4. I believe the emphasis on effective problem solving in this organization ranks   _____.

5. I believe the concern for the process of shared governance ranks   _____.

6. My level of satisfaction with this organization ranks   _____.

Any question you do not understand or do not have sufficient information to answer, please leave blank.

Part C: Demographics

1. My current role here is:
   - ❏ Staff nurse
   - ❏ Specialist (not a manager)
   - ❏ First line manager (responsible for one unit)
   - ❏ Other manager (responsible for more than one unit)
   - ❏ Senior manager (responsible for entire division)
   - ❏ Other _____.
2. My regular unit is _____.
3. My regular shift is _____.
4. I have worked this shift for ____ years.
5. I have worked for this organization for ___ years.
6. I work here primarily because: (Select only one.)
   - ❏ It is convenient.
   - ❏ Pay and benefits are good.
   - ❏ Satisfying work environment and relationships.
   - ❏ I have to work and this is as good a place as any.
   - ❏ I do not like working here.
   - ❏ Other _____.
7. If I left here it would be primarily because: (Select only one.)
   - ❏ I was offered a better job.
   - ❏ Better pay and benefits.
   - ❏ More work satisfaction.
   - ❏ I was unhappy working here.
   - ❏ Spousal transfer or domestic situation.
   - ❏ I need a change.
   - ❏ Other _____.

8. I typically work ___ hours per week.
9. My age is ___ years.
10. My highest level of formal education is: (Select only one.)
    - ❏ High school
    - ❏ Vocational or technical school
    - ❏ Community college program
    - ❏ Diploma program
    - ❏ University degree
    - ❏ Graduate degree
11. I am currently taking classes:
    - ❏ yes ❏ no (Select only one.)
    If yes, then please answer the following question: I am studying: _____.
12. I have participated or been involved in shared governance in the following ways:

    _____

    _____

13. If my involvement in shared governance has been minimal or not at all, it is because:

    _____

    _____

14. Please comment about this questionnaire. Feel free to include anything you think will improve it or will address you issues more fully:

    _____

    _____

15. If you feel an important question was not asked, please write it for us so that we might assess it for future preparation.

    _____

    _____

TOOL D: Survey of Shared Leadership Practices

Instructions: This is a survey of your manager's practices and whether or not she or he engages in behaviors that allow you to do your best work in a shared leadership organization. You may also use this tool to evaluate your council or shared decision making group leaders, as well as to facilitate the group to do its best work.

Managers and leaders in empowered organizations purposefully engage in behaviors that enable staff members to effectively meet their professional accountabilities. The items in this survey have been carefully selected as representative of these shared leadership practices. Please examine each scenario and reflect on how characteristic it is of your manager or group leader, by thinking about how frequently she or he engages in this behavior.

To the right of each scenario, you are asked to make two sets of ratings:

Actual: Your assessment of how frequently your manager is actually engaged in shared leadership behaviors.

Desired: Your assessment of how often, in order for you to meet your professional accountabilities, you would like your manager to be using a certain shared leadership practice.

Read each scenario and record both an actual and a desired assessment in the boxes located in the *right margin* of this survey.

Use the following scales in making your own assessments:

1. Always	5. Sometimes
2. Nearly always	6. Hardly ever
3. Frequently	7. Rarely
4. Half the Time	

Actual   ❑ ❑ ❑ ❑ ❑ ❑
Desired ❑ ❑ ❑ ❑ ❑ ❑

1 2 3 4 5 6 7

1. Actively seeks opportunities to help staff groups who are trying to achieve a goal. Eases groups through a process to accomplish goals. Remains neutral and helps the group stay focused.
   Actual   ❑ ❑ ❑ ❑ ❑ ❑
   Desired ❑ ❑ ❑ ❑ ❑ ❑

2. Recognizes that the work of groups is based on each staff member's attitudes, commitment, values, and skills. Enthusiastically works to bring these into the problem-solving process.
   Actual   ❑ ❑ ❑ ❑ ❑ ❑
   Desired ❑ ❑ ❑ ❑ ❑ ❑

3. Clearly spells out her or his won facilitator roles and responsibilities to shared leadership groups.
   Actual   ❑ ❑ ❑ ❑ ❑ ❑
   Desired ❑ ❑ ❑ ❑ ❑ ❑

4. Observes the various roles that group members play in groups, the methods that they use in decision making, and their communication patterns. Freely shares this information with the group to help them to work better together.
   Actual   ❑ ❑ ❑ ❑ ❑ ❑
   Desired ❑ ❑ ❑ ❑ ❑ ❑

5. Always protects individuals and their ideas from attack by other staff members. Through her or his own words and actions, communicates the dignity and the individual worth of each person and confidence in her/his ability to make a contribution.

Actual ❏ ❏ ❏ ❏ ❏ ❏ ❏
Desired ❏ ❏ ❏ ❏ ❏ ❏ ❏

6. Assists staff to develop their skills but does not direct or take responsibility for people's skill development. Encourages staff to try new ways of working without fear of failure.

Actual ❏ ❏ ❏ ❏ ❏ ❏ ❏
Desired ❏ ❏ ❏ ❏ ❏ ❏ ❏

7. Suggests to staff members the opportunities to expand their skills. Conveys to each person that her or his work is central to the success of this organization.

Actual ❏ ❏ ❏ ❏ ❏ ❏ ❏
Desired ❏ ❏ ❏ ❏ ❏ ❏ ❏

8. When coaching people, the manager's conversation makes sense, follows logic, and communicates that the manager is giving the staff her or his undivided attention.

Actual ❏ ❏ ❏ ❏ ❏ ❏ ❏
Desired ❏ ❏ ❏ ❏ ❏ ❏ ❏

9. Sets time aside to assist staff members and work groups to develop their skills. Is approachable and available when needed. Does not remain aloof.

Actual ❏ ❏ ❏ ❏ ❏ ❏ ❏
Desired ❏ ❏ ❏ ❏ ❏ ❏ ❏

10. Clearly communicates to staff members any performance problems. Focuses on solutions rather than problems. Does not become emotional or critical when confronting staff. Protects people's self-esteem when discussing performance problems.

Actual ❏ ❏ ❏ ❏ ❏ ❏ ❏
Desired ❏ ❏ ❏ ❏ ❏ ❏ ❏

11. Really listens to staff. Asks questions to clarify understanding of other people's points of view. Does not interrupt or let mind wander during conversations.

Actual ❏ ❏ ❏ ❏ ❏ ❏ ❏
Desired ❏ ❏ ❏ ❏ ❏ ❏ ❏

12. Stimulates reluctant staff members to participate by drawing them out and engaging them in active dialogue.

Actual ❏ ❏ ❏ ❏ ❏ ❏ ❏
Desired ❏ ❏ ❏ ❏ ❏ ❏ ❏

Dimension I ☐ **Total Score Actual**

☐ **Total Score Desired**

13. Works hard to gain support for her or his own ideas. Does not manipulate or withhold information to advance her or his own ideas.

Actual   ☐ ☐ ☐ ☐ ☐ ☐ ☐
Desired ☐ ☐ ☐ ☐ ☐ ☐ ☐

14. Spends little time worrying about what the "higher-ups" are thinking. Bravely represents people and groups, even if the issue is unpopular with senior management.

Actual   ☐ ☐ ☐ ☐ ☐ ☐ ☐
Desired ☐ ☐ ☐ ☐ ☐ ☐ ☐

15. Always puts people first. Is fair and consistent in treatment of others. Shows no favoritism. Helps people avoid conforming to social pressures at work.

Actual   ☐ ☐ ☐ ☐ ☐ ☐ ☐
Desired ☐ ☐ ☐ ☐ ☐ ☐ ☐

16. Can be counted on to follow up. Keeps commitments and is respected for honesty. People know what she or he believes.

Actual   ☐ ☐ ☐ ☐ ☐ ☐ ☐
Desired ☐ ☐ ☐ ☐ ☐ ☐ ☐

17. Solicits feedback about impact on others. Responds nondefensively to criticism about her or his own actions.

Actual   ☐ ☐ ☐ ☐ ☐ ☐ ☐
Desired ☐ ☐ ☐ ☐ ☐ ☐ ☐

18. Communicates a leadership vision in a way that inspires others to act. Has a strong sense of purpose. Can describe how her or his own work and the work of others contribute to the achievement of the organization's mission.

Actual   ☐ ☐ ☐ ☐ ☐ ☐ ☐
Desired ☐ ☐ ☐ ☐ ☐ ☐ ☐

19. Communicates self-respect and personal commitment to doing the best job possible. Openly works to resolve staff difficulties with her or his leadership style.

Actual   ☐ ☐ ☐ ☐ ☐ ☐ ☐
Desired ☐ ☐ ☐ ☐ ☐ ☐ ☐

20. Sees power as available to everyone rather than a limited resource. Assumes that staff members are accountable, with the necessary freedom and authority to do their work. Affirms the personal power of each individual.

Actual   ☐ ☐ ☐ ☐ ☐ ☐ ☐
Desired ☐ ☐ ☐ ☐ ☐ ☐ ☐

21. Frees staff members to collaborate and share in decision making. Gets staff personally involved in the work to be done. Accepts staff's control of the content and pace of their own work.

Actual   ☐ ☐ ☐ ☐ ☐ ☐ ☐
Desired ☐ ☐ ☐ ☐ ☐ ☐ ☐

22. Works hard to eliminate policies, procedures, or systems that interfere with getting the job done.

Actual   ☐ ☐ ☐ ☐ ☐ ☐ ☐
Desired ☐ ☐ ☐ ☐ ☐ ☐ ☐

23. Translates the principles of empowerment to staff through role-modeling and fulfilling expectations of staff decision-making groups.

Actual   ☐ ☐ ☐ ☐ ☐ ☐ ☐
Desired ☐ ☐ ☐ ☐ ☐ ☐ ☐

24. Questions staff members regularly regarding their understanding and participation in empowerment activities.

Actual   ☐ ☐ ☐ ☐ ☐ ☐ ☐
Desired ☐ ☐ ☐ ☐ ☐ ☐ ☐

Dimension II ☐ **Total Score Actual**

☐ **Total Score Desired**

57

25. Communicates to everyone well-defined and clear goals for change. Freely provides information for the duration of change.

Actual ❑ ❑ ❑ ❑ ❑ ❑ ❑
Desired ❑ ❑ ❑ ❑ ❑ ❑ ❑

26. Establishes and then coaches staff work groups to manage the changes that affect their work.

Actual ❑ ❑ ❑ ❑ ❑ ❑ ❑
Desired ❑ ❑ ❑ ❑ ❑ ❑ ❑

27. Ensures that change is not disconnected from organizational realities by obtaining the necessary commitment, people, materials, and financial support before embarking on change.

Actual ❑ ❑ ❑ ❑ ❑ ❑ ❑
Desired ❑ ❑ ❑ ❑ ❑ ❑ ❑

28. Assists staff in using project management processes to set timelines, allocate resources, prioritize actions, and assign responsibilities.

Actual ❑ ❑ ❑ ❑ ❑ ❑ ❑
Desired ❑ ❑ ❑ ❑ ❑ ❑ ❑

29. Helps staff identify specific and measurable outcomes to track successes and failures. Sees failures as opportunities for learning. Facilities staff's progress in evaluating themselves and unit outcomes.

Actual ❑ ❑ ❑ ❑ ❑ ❑ ❑
Desired ❑ ❑ ❑ ❑ ❑ ❑ ❑

30. Acts consistently on the belief that every person helps design her or his own work. Instead of informing people of a better way to do their jobs, staff members are coached by the manager to invent their jobs themselves.

Actual ❑ ❑ ❑ ❑ ❑ ❑ ❑
Desired ❑ ❑ ❑ ❑ ❑ ❑ ❑

31. Re-thinks work from the customer's focus. Helps staff design systems of work that are flexible, reflect what customers desire, and provide meaningful work for each person that is cost-effective.

Actual ❑ ❑ ❑ ❑ ❑ ❑ ❑
Desired ❑ ❑ ❑ ❑ ❑ ❑ ❑

32. Encourages staff on different units, departments, or different shifts to organize their work differently, depending on skill mix, people availability, and so on. Recognizes that there is more than one way to "skin a cat."

Actual ❑ ❑ ❑ ❑ ❑ ❑ ❑
Desired ❑ ❑ ❑ ❑ ❑ ❑ ❑

33. Avoids rigid or fixed ways of doing work. As conditions change, helps the staff re-invent the way work is performed as they learn and as the world changes.

Actual ❑ ❑ ❑ ❑ ❑ ❑ ❑
Desired ❑ ❑ ❑ ❑ ❑ ❑ ❑

34. Confronts negative staff members with the truth about changes in work expectations and empowerment activities.

Actual ❑ ❑ ❑ ❑ ❑ ❑ ❑
Desired ❑ ❑ ❑ ❑ ❑ ❑ ❑

Dimension III ❑ **Total Score Actual**
❑ **Total Score Desired**

35. Directly addresses objections to participation in decision making, countering staff members' objections to participation in decision making.

Actual ❑❑❑❑❑❑❑
Desired ❑❑❑❑❑❑❑

36. Staff decision-making meetings are held at least monthly to deal with staff accountability issues.

Actual ❑❑❑❑❑❑❑
Desired ❑❑❑❑❑❑❑

37. Provides staff members access to information, resources, and time, at least weekly, regarding organizational changes. Asks for response and feedback from staff.

Actual ❑❑❑❑❑❑❑
Desired ❑❑❑❑❑❑❑

38. Incorporates people from every staff role into discussions about patient care and staff work.

Actual ❑❑❑❑❑❑❑
Desired ❑❑❑❑❑❑❑

39. Communicates budget and financial information regularly to the staff. Keeps them informed about changes in finance affecting their work and lives.

Actual ❑❑❑❑❑❑❑
Desired ❑❑❑❑❑❑❑

40. Always helps the staff include financial or resource components in every decision.

Actual ❑❑❑❑❑❑❑
Desired ❑❑❑❑❑❑❑

41. Provides staff members with the time to attend staff decision-making group meetings. Actively and enthusiastically embraces their participation in staff decisions.

Actual ❑❑❑❑❑❑❑
Desired ❑❑❑❑❑❑❑

42. Shares with staff her or his own accountabilities and performance expectations as a manager. Seeks feedback regarding leadership performance.

Actual ❑❑❑❑❑❑❑
Desired ❑❑❑❑❑❑❑

43. Communicates activities, concerns, manager's role, and issues with the medical staff. Has an ongoing and regular pattern of communication with doctors.

Actual ❑❑❑❑❑❑❑
Desired ❑❑❑❑❑❑❑

44. Creates an environment where staff feel connected to their manager and feel great working with and relating to her or him.

Actual ❑❑❑❑❑❑❑
Desired ❑❑❑❑❑❑❑

45. Unit runs well. Staff and management generally relate well. Together, they confront change positively, with good results.

Actual ❑❑❑❑❑❑❑
Desired ❑❑❑❑❑❑❑

Dimension IV ❑ **Total Score Actual**

❑ **Total Score Desired**

Instructions for Scoring Your Self-Assessment of Shared Leadership Practices

Part I

The self-assessment of *Shared Leadership Practices* assesses your managerial or leadership practices along four core Dimensions, and whether or not they are productive. A total score for the survey can be computed as well as a separate score for each Dimension.

1. Please total the scores on your self assessment for each component, and place in the box below.
2. Add your Dimension scores together to get a total score.

Dimension I ☐
Facilitating and Coaching

Dimension II ☐
Empowerment

Dimension III ☐
Change Management

Dimension IV ☐
Shared Leadership
Principles

TOTAL I-IV ☐

Instructions for Scoring Part II

1. Now total the performance scores from your staff survey.
2. Record your self assessment scores from the previous page in the appropriate box below.
3. For each Dimension, add together the staff actual scores for all of your staff surveys. Divide this number by the numbers of surveys returned. Enter the mean score in the appropriate box below. Repeat this exercise for the staff desired scores.
4. Record total scores by adding the Dimension scores you had recorded in the previous steps.

	My Self Assessment	Staff Actual	Staff Desired
Dimension I Facilitating and Coaching	☐	☐	☐
Dimension II Empowerment	☐	☐	☐
Dimension III Change Management	☐	☐	☐
Dimension IV Shared Leadership Principles	☐	☐	☐
MY TOTAL SCORES **Dimension I-IV**	☐	☐	☐

HOW DOES MY STAFF FEEDBACK COMPARE WITH MY SELF-ASSESSMENT OF MY FACILITATION AND MY COACHING SKILLS?

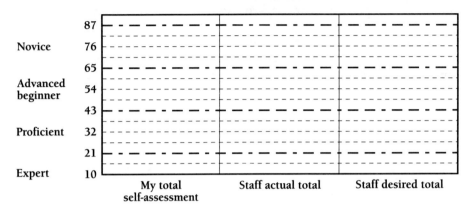

Instructions: Plot your *Self, Staff actual,* and *Staff desired* scores for **Dimension I** on the graph.

HOW DOES MY STAFF FEEDBACK COMPARE WITH MY SELF-ASSESSMENT OF MY EMPOWERMENT SKILLS?

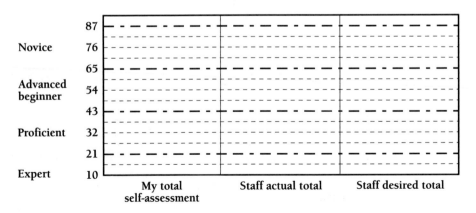

Instructions: Plot your *Self, Staff actual,* and *Staff desired* scores for **Dimension II** on the graph.

HOW DOES MY STAFF FEEDBACK COMPARE WITH MY SELF-ASSESSMENT OF MY APPROACH TO CHANGE?

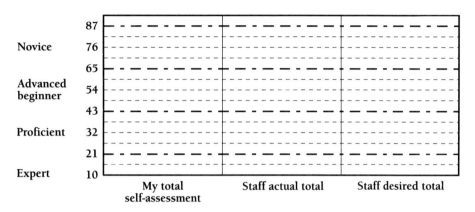

Instructions: Plot your *Self, Staff actual,* and *Staff desired* scores for **Dimension III** on the graph.

HOW DOES MY STAFF FEEDBACK COMPARE WITH MY SELF-ASSESSMENT OF MY APPLICATION OF SHARED LEADERSHIP PRINCIPLES?

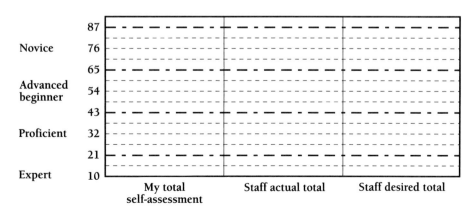

Instructions: Plot your *Self, Staff actual,* and *Staff desired* scores for **Dimension IV** on the graph.

HOW DOES MY STAFF FEEDBACK COMPARE WITH MY SELF-ASSESSMENT OF SHARED LEADERSHIP PRINCIPLES?

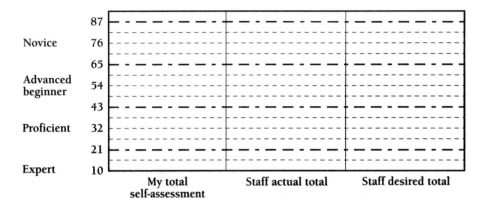

Instructions: Plot your overall *Self-assessment, Total staff actual,* and *Staff desired* scores on the graph.

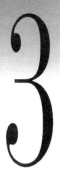

Getting Started with Teams

*Ideas must work through the brains and arms of people
or they are no better than dreams.*

Ralph Waldo Emerson

THE BASIC COMPONENTS OF TEAM BUILDING

Health care teams are different, both in the nature of the groups and the content of their work. Because patients depend specifically on the knowledge, understanding, and interface of all team members in their progress along the continuum of care, the knowledge, relationships, and integration of the activities of the team become critical in providing health care services. Therefore the construction of the team is an important process that should be approached carefully and critically.

Many kinds of teams can be constructed, including quality teams, project teams, goal teams, process teams, and improvement teams; however, almost all effective teams have common elements. The focus of this chapter will be on the health care team at the point of service. The health care component is specifically identified because of the nature of the service provided.

THE FOUNDATION OF ALL TEAMS

Every team has basic components and constructs that define it. Every team must undergo certain processes to build the activities associated with the

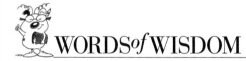

WORDS*of*WISDOM

There are all kinds of teams, but they all have common characteristics that are central to their success. Forget these elements and you have no team.

~

BOX 3-1

Elements for an Effective Team

There are common elements in the construction of an effective team. These must be the focus of development at the outset of setting up the team:
- Purpose
- Goals
- Roles
- Relationships
- Activities and functions
- Coordination and leadership

Every team is simply the aggregation of the skills, talents, and behaviors of its participants. It is critical that the roles of all team members be clear and understood at the outset. It is ambiguity around role that can create the largest number of difficulties.

team (Box 3-1). The following elements are essential to the construction of any team and should be a part of the work of leadership in initiating activities around teams.

Essential Elements for Team Construction

Purpose

Every team must have a purpose for its existence and a direction to its work. In clinical teams, the purpose is to organize differentiated and distributed practitioners around a common goal with common processes associated with delivering patient care. Therefore the purpose of the team is to configure the workers in a meaningful way to support the delivery of patient care.

Goals

Every team, subsequent to defining its purpose, has specific goals that fulfill that purpose. The goal of clinical teams is to configure providers in a unique arrangement around patient processes to meet the demands of patient care. These goals specifically enumerate the character and content of the role of the team and ultimately its members.

Roles

Every clinical team has members whose role best ensures that the functions and activities of the team will be carried out consistent with its purposes. No two teams are alike. The service that is provided, the patient population that is served, and the various players that make up the team create the unique character of the team. Each individual role, when joined with all roles, creates the team framework that ensures the team meets its purposes and the needs of those it serves. Each individual role must be clearly defined within its own context, as well as in relationship to the aggregated roles of all members of the team. Role clarity becomes one of the basic requisites of an effective team.

In health care teams focus on accountability becomes a critical part of the expectation of individual roles. Each team member is accountable for some specific outcome. Other team members depend on the proper performance of the roles, functions, activities, and responsibilities associated with a team member's accountability for their work to be successful. As with all teams, it is the aggregated function of team members converging their efforts that creates the foundation for successful team outcomes. Clear roles is one of the centerpieces of building effective teams.

Relationships

No team can operate successfully or be sustained without a clear set of relationships and an effective interaction between team members. The effectiveness of team roles is not achieved by accident. The studied, well defined, clearly integrated process of relationship building and ensuring the maintenance of good relationships is an ongoing, functional part of teams. Clinical teams require a special focus on relationships because much of the work that is involved depends on the contribution of each team member to the process of delivering patient care services for a range of patients with a number of other providers (Box 3-2). Each role depends on the proficiency, effectiveness, and relatedness of other roles on the team. Building solid, open, honest, and meaningful relationships becomes a critical part of sustaining the team's activities and building the trust necessary for the work of the team to be effective. The expectation of both the patient and the organization around teams is that the outcomes of the teams are consistently achieved and maintained. Therefore it is the expectation of the team that the relationships necessary to continue to focus on appropriate team outcomes be consistently and continuously configured in a way that advances the work of the team and meets the obligation of the team for its outcomes.

Teams depend on the kind of relationship the members are able to establish with each other. It is critical to the team's life that issues of personality, behavior, and style be on the agenda and discussed if congruence is to be present in the team.

BOX **3-2**

Characteristics of Clinical Teams
Clinical teams are unique and have special characteristics: 1. Their focus is on the patient rather than the team. 2. The outcomes of work are less easy to measure. 3. Each team member has his or her own disciplinary considerations. 4. The team's goal is to get the patient to rely less on the team.

Activities and functions

All teams, of course, have specific activities that must be accomplished for the team's work to get done. The negotiated and expected components of individual roles must converge in way that meets the team's needs and ensures that the purposes and the outcomes of the team are achieved. Each team member has a set of activities and functions that will be necessary to the performance of his or her role. Each of these activities and functions must be configured in a way that supports, facilitates, yet does not duplicate the role of others. To get to that level of efficiency, a good deal of dialogue will be undertaken to assure that there is a clarity around the various functions and activities each of the members of the team will perform. Of course, there are issues of competence, skill, appropriateness, distribution, and other elements of individual functions and activities that must be negotiated between the players. In multidisciplinary care teams it becomes increasingly important to determine which provider will undertake what activities. This is so because some providers are able to perform many of the same activities and, through development and refocusing of activities and functions, may even be cross-trained to perform activities not previously considered a part of their role. All of the issues associated with this should be clarified by the participants from the team to make sure that there is a good fit between and among the various functions and activities of each member of the team.

Coordination and leadership

All teams need to have a clear sense of direction and have an obligation to fulfill the purposes to which they were constructed. Therefore the team efforts and activities need to be coordinated and some leadership needs to be provided in a way that helps the team focus on its own issues, as well as its concerns around productivity, performance, expectation, evaluation, conflict, and the maintaining of outcomes. Even in the arena of self-managed work teams the coordination and integration of activities becomes an important part of the effectiveness and sustenance of the individual team. Although leadership and coordination in self-directed work teams may not

The clinical team's work is defined by the culture and circumstances of each patient it serves. There is no standard operating procedure that does not have to be modified in some way to meet the unique needs of each patient. That is what makes clinical teams different.

Leadership is not management in team-based systems. Most leadership must now be provided by clinicians at the point-of-service. There is a growing demand for real staff leaders.

always be undertaken by the same individual, various activities around team effectiveness will require certain lead functions consistent with the team role (Team Tip 3-1). For example, the collection of data, evaluation of process, coordination of team dynamics, meeting processes, conflict resolution, and performance evaluation all require some level of coordination and leadership. Each team, of course, will have to work out for itself based on the approach to building teams as to how that leadership is provided. In some teams that leadership is designated and defined by the organization. In some it is identified by the team. In others it is coordinated and rotated among the various members of the team based on skill, role, and expectation. It is critical that all of the issues around team leadership be identified as early in the process of building teams as possible.

PITFALLS TO AVOID WHEN INITIATING TEAMS

There is a lot of mythology and fable around the issue of building effective teams. Although there is much work and literature on effective team building over time in the implementation of team approaches, some indicators of effectiveness and ineffectiveness have emerged. Through the past decade and a half in the team-building process those elements that work and those that do not have been identified. The initiation of teams should require a careful study of the risks involved in team-based approaches and critical process and considerations developed around those elements that work and those that do not. Some of the critical risks should be considered at the outset.

Team Fables

Fable one: team members always feel committed to implementing a team process

This fable states a myth that is most dangerous. Most people in the clinical frame of reference, while they have worked with each other, have not necessarily worked with each other in a team framework. Working in the same place, in the same department, and with the same patients does not

TEAMTIP 3.1

Team Leadership Needs
Leaders always need data to lead. In team leadership the needs are:
• Rules of behavior
• Patient information
• Financial data
• Clinical protocols
• Clinical roles of members
• Work assignment patterns
• Support systems

Fables about teams and team building abound. The truth about team formation is often not so much what people desire but what they do. People may want successful teams, but they may not want to make the changes or do the work that is required.

WORDS*of*WISDOM

Working with others is a learned skill. No matter how we know other team members, working in the context of team requires a higher level of interaction and relationship. Building that relationship will be work!

~

Everyone brings something different to the team. Members should not expect that they will easily accommodate the behaviors and talents of others. Adaptation processes will be necessary to create comfort with personal and work style differences.

guarantee that people are working in teams. Building a team-based construct for undertaking clinical work is different from simply doing clinical work with other people. Also, one should not be deluded into believing that people really want to work as teams. Most people do not know how to work within the context of teams. It is a learned skill. Given time, a good implementation process, and a carefully constructed approach to team building, they will learn. However, team construction should not be initiated with the belief that people are able to or even want to operate effectively as team members.

Fable two: all team members are created equal

This is perhaps one of the most dangerous considerations in building teams. Team members come to the role of team interaction believing different things about the contribution, interaction, and relationship of other members in the team. Therefore there are some real concerns around the issues of equity, balance, and involvement of members in a team. The physician clearly comes to the team with a different perception than does the respiratory therapist. The nurse comes with a different understanding of her or his role than does the physical therapist or nutritionist. Each member comes with a set of insights, precepts, and levels of understanding regarding his or her role in the function of the team that must be clarified and ascertained at the outset. Much of the developmental processes associated with the team will be working through the inequity of perception or role that people bring to the team process.

Fable three: people can reach agreement on their issues of concern

Perhaps one of the most difficult components of building effective teams is decision making and creating consensus around meaningful decision making. Many people do not know how to make good group decisions. They do not understand the process of consensus building or recognize that consensus can be obtained through the use of appropriate techniques and methodology. However, knowing these techniques will be critical to the effectiveness of decision making on the team. Learning the processes will be important to the success of the team in its own problem solving. However, this learning is a process, and therefore much effort must be devoted to the activities associated with building skill, insight, and ability around techniques and methodology.

Fable four: team members will use critical thinking to resolve problems and issues

One of the most disheartening processes of team building is the recognition that the team members do not necessarily exhibit the skills they are assumed to have. Analytical, objective, deductive, or reductive processes are not often used in the process of doing work. Much of the skill that is reflected in the rendering of patient services is intuitive, a reflection of the talents and skills obtained over time that are almost second nature to the practitioner. In team-based activities, these processes must be made visible to other team members in logical and organized ways. This is not necessarily exciting work, nor is it easy to do in a way that can transfer to others the skill and insights around the activities carried out by an individual team member. However, as difficult as this process may be, it is an important part of the functional activities of the team. Therefore developing the skills necessary to articulate functions, activities, practices, and priorities; translating these skills in language that can be understood by team members; and implementing processes that have logic, analysis, and rationale will become an important part of the team construction process.

Fable five: people will set their emotions aside in the interest of the team

It is an ideal expectation that people are able to balance their emotions against the requirements of the team, but this usually does not happen at the outset. Again, such balance is a learned skill and requires some focus and developmental activity on the part of the team. Team facilitation should include a studied and careful dialogue around the issue of emotion,

Finding common ground is not simple work. However, once practice with good methodology bears fruit it can become easy and routine. Faithfulness to the process will be necessary to maintain good skills and high levels of consensus.

Skill development is the continuous work of the team. Like the rest of the organization, team members are perceptual learners. Assumptions should never be made about critical thinking skills. There is always more to learn in refining critical problem-solving skills.

Team members bring all their strengths and flaws into the team with them. Working to build good relationships means dealing with the whole package as it is.

Each of us develop our patterns of behavior over the years of our lives. It is a false expectation that we always know why we do what we do. Careful and caring attention to addressing the habits and rituals of others is important to building community. Good technique and method can make the process work and create an effective framework for addressing delicate personal issues affecting team function.

feeling, expression, and team membership. It must be remembered that it is people who make up teams and that individuals on teams bring with them all of the elements and processes that define them as individuals. Simply becoming a member of the team does not shift the individual characteristics and behaviors that people bring to the team. Discussing the implications of the feelings, emotions, relationships, and sense of membership on the team is a part of the process of building a team; therefore it should be a part of the initial work of building teams.

Fable six: each of us know why we do what we do

One of the mysteries of relationships is recognizing that people bring different meaning, value, and insights to their activity and their relationships. Some of that is done unconsciously. Therefore the impact of an individual's behavior on another may not be discerned by the individual because of the normalcy of the behavior to the originating party and the lack of insight around the unique impact it might have on another person. We all make assumptions about our behaviors. We all behave in ways that we do not necessarily consciously consider in advance of the behavior. Clearly, however, these behaviors can have an impact on others who are assessing the impact of our behaviors on them. There must be space in team development where these unconscious processes, activities, behaviors, and notions have a way of being worked out, identified, and laid on the table in a way that is meaningful to the participants. The discernment process makes obvious those things that may be of concern to others while they may not necessarily be a part of our conscious and individual awareness. Dialogue between team members does the most to create the milieu for dealing with these differences.

Fable seven: people really want to work together

The truth is that people do not necessarily want or know how to work together. Most of the work in the past has been individually assigned work to each member of the group. Such group work is not the same as teamwork. Recognizing that the constructs of teams and that the elements of work in relationship to building teams is different from simply working in groups becomes a critical part of the team-building process. People do not necessarily know how teamwork operates—how to become an integrated, tightly fitted, continuous, and synergistic member of a team. Although synergy may be the outcome of good teamwork, it is not achieved quickly, nor is it effected easily. The achievement of synergy can only come over time. Building toward it will require careful, day-to-day relationship and interaction building work using continuous methods and skills that can result in effective relationships. Assuming that this is possible without doing the necessary work will not result in an effective and cohesive team.

Fable eight: teams will grow naturally

The truth is, teams do not grow naturally. Teams are not consistently continuous and contiguous processes to develop. Teams, like much of life, grow intermittently, with pushes and pulls, ups and downs, flurries of activity and periods of dormancy. The incremental and intermittent processes associated with team development represent the highly variable nature of relationships that often exist between individuals and in groups. Therefore it should not be expected that the team process and its development will flow in a seamless, continuous process through concerted and integrated activities. Like all human dynamics, there will be a series of processes, functions, and activities that will emerge at different rates depending on the maturity, character, and issues with which the team is concerned. It should be anticipated that there will be varying degrees of intensity within the process of team building that will affect the rate and the pace of constructing effective teams.

Fable nine: trust building is an important part of team building

The truth is, trust is not something that can be built. Trust is actually evidence of what is already in place. Trust is the visible representation of the work already done in building relationships between team members and

Not everyone is comfortable or even knows how to work in teams. Some people have always "gone it alone." Building opportunity to manage in one's own space will need to be balanced against the requirements of team performance. Seeking this balance will require some experimentation with team and personal boundary setting.

The process of working together has always been an expectation of work. The techniques of working together have not always been available. To make it happen the techniques must be applied and reinforced.

Trust is not something anyone can create. Trust is evidence of what is already in place. If there is an effective, well-functioning team with confidence and good relationships, trust will always be present.

In the past we have been great at focusing on good process. It is only recently that outcome measurement has become a critical part of our work. It will require new learning and a change in focus to become good at achieving and replicating consistent outcomes.

creating effectiveness around teams. Therefore trust is evidence rather than circumstance. We cannot build trust; we can only undertake the activities that result in a sense of trust between and among the members. It is important to recognize that building the elements that will result in trust is a continuous and ongoing process that never stops. Trust can be broken through one major breach of relationship or through a series of minor breaks in the relationships between and among team members. The constant effort of a team is not so much in building trust but in generating relationships, processes, and methodologies that get at those issues on which trust depends: strong relationships, the ability to problem solve, skill in dealing with individual performance issues, and the group's ability to consistently obtain group outcomes. Attention to each of these will be critical to the maintenance of trust and the advancing of the group's collective identity.

Fable ten: group members will continuously focus on the outcomes to which their work is directed

Group members will not always focus on the outcomes to which their work is directed. Indeed, sometimes group members will not be clear about what those activities are that facilitate continuous outcome. A part of the functional work of the team is to determine consistently what outcomes are of value and how work can be directed toward consistently obtaining those outcomes. Evaluating outcome (and the requirements necessary to obtain it) is one of the purposes of a team. Outcomes change when performance expectations are adjusted. When specific outcomes have been obtained for a long period of time, it may be a sign that it is time to change the outcome, raise the standard, or advance the expectation. Each of these conditions and circumstances has an influence on the value, purpose, and meaning of the work of the team and therefore must be continually refocused and reemphasized as a part of the evaluative process of teams. It often occurs in the workplace that people get so tied up in their activities and functions that they often forget the purpose of those processes. When the work becomes an end in itself, the purpose and meaning of the work are often lost. Reacquainting team members with such purposes and outcomes helps reaffirm and firmly establish the meaning and value to which individual work and teamwork is directed.

Although these risks do not identify all of the areas of concern around the development of teams, they highlight some of the main issues around creating effective teams. Other risks must be identified as well, around the role of facilitation, leadership activities and functions, team perceptions and commitment, decision-making processes and techniques, and a host of other issues that are a part of the functional activities associated with building effective teams. As with most of these activities, team building becomes a constant and consistent process and requires a widely variable degree of intensity and attention depending on the issues, the maturity, and the conditions that affect the kind and character of the work of the team.

THE PRIMARY PHASES OF TEAM BUILDING

Teams, like any other dynamic in life, have specific phases through which they move on the way to maturity and continuity. Primary phases of team development indicate the specific changes that the team goes through as it becomes more fully integrated and functional.

Focus on Purpose

In the beginning phase the team focuses essentially on its purpose, the establishment of parameters and guidelines for movement toward the process of being a team. In this phase the first steps relate specifically to structuring the goals, direction, purpose, and meaning of the team as a fundamental part of its first-stage activities.

In creating the direction for the team, some of the first activities relate to outlining the steps and processes associated with becoming a team. Initially the team's purpose must be articulated in a way that each member can understand (Box 3-3). Out of that particular direction must come a focus on looking at the specific elements of the team that give it meaning and form. Questions related to those activities include the following:

Building team-based organizations is a high-risk activity. Although people may have worked together, they may not have a relationship with each other around mutual expectations. To build that relationship takes time and work.

BOX **3-3**

Constructing Purpose
• Keep the purpose simple.
• Make sure the purpose meets the mission of the system.
• Ensure that the purpose is clear to all who read it.
• Make sure the purpose gives clear direction.
• Ensure that the purpose reflects the meaning behind the activities it directs.

The team's purpose should always be clear and simple. The participants should avoid high-sounding terminology and devise a clear and simple message supporting their work and goals.

TEAM**TIP**   3.2

Constructing Priorities

Team members, to be thorough, often construct more priorities than they will ever be able to address. There should be no more than three to five priorities around which work activities will be centered. This ensures that the goals can actually be accomplished.

Each team member must make a contribution to the work of the team. Each should be clear about what that is. In teams everyone is responsible for achieving the teams outcomes. Goals are therefore personal commitments to the team's work.

- What contribution to the activities of the organization will the team make?
- How will the team focus on the functions of patient care?
- What is different about working as a team rather than as individuals?

Once these and related questions are asked, the team's purpose should be clearly drafted and outlined as a foundation for determining the team's work. Once the purpose has been clearly articulated, the team members can begin to establish a foundation on which they will build their own activities. This becomes a critical subset of the work the team has in undertaking formation of the initial steps of becoming an integrated work group.

Developing Goals and Priorities

As the team begins to understand its purpose and the direction that it has in the organization, it now must be clear about what specific objectives or goals will fulfill its purposes. The team has chosen the direction that it will take and has outlined clearly in its purpose what its meaning is and its value in the organizational system. Now the team must be clear about what its actions and activities will be based on as a way of giving direction and focus to the team (Team Tip 3-2).

Questions that relate specifically to obtaining focus should form the center of the activities of the team in its goal-defining function—questions around individual team member contribution, specific and defined goals and direction for the organization, processes associated with reaching those goals, measurable elements that outline the identifiers around the goals, a clearer set of indications that give form to those goals, and a clearer understanding of the team's central commitment to obtaining the goals and direction that it has established. Each of these elements forms the foundation for the processes related to team building and the activities that evidence the initial stage of team construction. Clearly, involved in all of these will be issues around the team's identification with each other, commitment to the process of building teams, resolution of differences, identification of conflicts, and other things that might give evidence of some initial challenges affecting the team's ability to take form or set direction.

THE PHASES OF TEAM BUILDING
Phase I: Establishing the Rules

Each team must have a set of rules or terms of engagement that identify the parameters within which the team operates (Box 3-4). These terms of reference become the framework that guides or disciplines the team's activities and functions, as well as the team members' relationships with each other. These rules of process help ensure that every team member has a clear understanding of his or her obligation to the team, to each other, and to his or her own role as a part of fulfilling the obligations of the team. The rules also discuss how the team works, relates, and interacts and the values and meaning that each member will bring to the process of problem resolutions, solution seeking, and goal fulfillment to which each is committed. All of these relate to membership, meeting attendance, timeliness, participation, contribution, and processes around problem solving and dealing with the issues of the team. These rules should relate to specific requirements for meeting attendance, the respect and trust each will show for the other, the formation of the requirements of participation, the expectations and obligations of team members, the commitments the team will have to its goals and purposes, the processes associated with decision making, and the mechanisms devoted to conflict resolution and solution seeking.

These steps form the foundation of the first stage of formation for team construction. Each team must have a framework within which it will operate and a set of rules around which it agrees to function and to interact as members of the team. These form the base on which subsequent work in team building will unfold and build for purposes of meeting the team's requirements in the organization.

Phase II: Team Clarification

Following the initial formative definitive stage of the team comes the processes associated with clarifying the functions, activities, relationships, and outcomes of the team. It is important for each team member to know what her or his contribution is to the team, the team's requirement for her or his role, the aggregated expectations of the team for its functions and ac-

BOX **3-4**

Rules of Engagement

Meeting times
Participation
Timeliness
Agenda
Business process
Dialogue
Member obligations
Discipline
Enforcement

Each member of the team needs to know what the team is all about. Therefore the team must clarify:
- *Functions*
- *Activities*
- *Relationships*
- *Interaction*
- *Processes*
- *Expectations*
- *Outcomes*

Teams need to be differentiated from each other to ensure a clear identity for the members. The uniqueness of the team is as important to its members as is the work it does. Allowing a way to create identity will be important to team cohesiveness.

BOX 3-5

Team Role Identity

Three role identity problems:
1. Unclear role definitions
2. Uncertain role functions
3. Undefined relationships

Three role identity solutions:
1. Specific role descriptions
2. Identification of role expectations
3. Process for role and relationship conflict resolution

tivities, and the requirements that will be essential to ensure that the team remains effective. Issues of team leadership, team responsibility, communication, and intersection with the organizational system and other teams become an important part of clarifying the team's functions and its roles. Through clarification of roles and responsibilities the team has an idea of what it can expect of members and what is necessary for team success.

What is critical is to make sure the team knows not only who it is, but what it does, as well as what it achieves through its own actions. Clarifying roles that are specific to the team helps the team identify itself more critically in relationship to expectation. Also, through the clarification process, elimination of duplication, overlapping expectations and responsibilities, gaps in role and function, and the failure to meet requirements and commitments can all be identified early in the process (Box 3-5). Each of these will help the team function better. Furthermore, clarification of team roles and functions and relationships helps the team gain a deeper understanding of the unique contribution each member can lend to the team's process. Certainly, every member of the team will bring something different. Looking at the different gifts and skills that team members have to offer, clarifying that in terms of how it fits the whole, will be important as a part of the process of determining the effectiveness of the team and the team's own commitment to its outcomes.

To be clear about the work and effectiveness of clarification, teams will have to be involved across the board. All team members should come to understand, as we identified in Chapters 1 and 2, that they are a part of a larger system, that they are members of the system, and that as members they have an obligation to fully participate. That participation should require that they express themselves, that they be called on to express for those who are quiet and more reflective in their approach, that they identify the specifics and the concerns that they have as team members, and that they address the specific performance expectations and their contribution to the team's accountabilities for the fulfillment of its goals and objectives. Involving all team members means developing methods and mechanisms for ensuring that all levels of communication are invested in the team's activities (Box 3-6). As with all human groups there are those who are dynamic, outgoing, and very articulate in their contribution. There are others who are more reflective, less articulate, but have as much to share and need to be called on to ensure that what they have to share is communicated. This means that the dynamics and processes of the initial phases of the team must include ways in which all members are involved in the communication and dialogue of the team around its expectations and roles.

To ensure that the team is specifically effective around those issues that are of direct concern to it, the team must be clear about its expectations and desires. The team must be able to know exactly what its assignments and functions will be, specifically in relationship to critical paths, patient care processes, and the activities of relationship of each team member to the others. Identifying specifics means being clear and detailed about the tasks, responsibilities, activities, and functions that each team member will bring to the process. When the team has clarified its expectations, those specifics of each team member must tie in to the expectations and goals the team has set for itself. The functions and activities of each team member, therefore, must in some way represent that member's particular contribution to fulfilling those expectations and accountabilities of the team as a whole.

Defining accountabilities

In team-based work, accountability is a critical element of the team's viability and function. Accountability is one of the central components of the whole process of integrated team-based organizational approaches. Accountability is the foundation of performance in the new organization. Unlike responsibility, which focuses on process effectiveness, accountability focuses on outcomes. The achievement of sustainable outcomes is the chief value of the work of the health system, and all members must be committed to that goal. As identified in Chapter 1, accountability is one of the four

---

BOX **3-6**

Involving Team Members

Involving all team members requires a method of deliberation that can be used throughout the work processes:
1. Format for deliberation that makes sense to the participants
2. Consistent use of the format in specific problem processes
3. Highlighting priority or pivotal problems for first review

Much of the initial work of the team is in setting common goals and expectations. Because of the diversity of the team's members, a good process for consensus building is necessary for team effectiveness.

BOX 3-7

Three Stages Of Accountability

Stage 1

Clarity: Each person must know how her or his work relates to the goals of the team.

Stage 2

Specificity: No generalizations are acceptable; each role must be specifically enumerated in relationship to team functions.

Stage 3

Outcomes: All team members must know their unique role and contribution to the achievement of results.

principles that are critical to the effectiveness, sustenance, and success of the organizational system. Accountability must be clearly articulated for each role. Certainly, there is the team's accountability for the clinical outcomes to which the team is directed. Each role, however, performs a specific set of functions and activities, which, when aggregated with others, contributes to the overall outcomes of the team's work. Therefore most of the work of accountability is individualized. Each member of the team, from therapist to nurse to physician must clearly articulate the contribution she or he makes to the team's functions, its relationship, work, and to the outcomes that the team has obligation to achieve. In this way all of the team members can look critically not only at their own expectations and accountabilities, but those of others, and make judgments about how they fit, work together, and, when aggregated, meet the needs of the team in achieving its clinical processes and the outcomes that reflect it.

Being clear about accountability is one of the most important critical elements upon which team success is built (Box 3-7). Therefore as much attention, energy, and activity as is necessary to be clear about that accountability should be undertaken. Furthermore, it would be appropriate for all members of the team to approach their accountability as a contract with each other and the organization such that all team members and the organization can expect the individual team members to fulfill the obligations associated with their accountability as they unfold the process of deliberation.

Accepting challenges

The formation of teams is not without its challenges. There will be opportunities for success as well as major barriers to the maintenance of team function and the obtaining of success. There will be a number of issues, personal as well as group, that will have to be addressed to make sure that team development continues to unfold as it should.

These challenges come in all kinds of formats (Box 3-8). They will be arrayed across the relationship-building process and in every element of team formation. Challenges will be faced regarding personal agendas; group process; individual communication styles; the kinds of issues and concerns that are communicated; circumstances around personal membership and the obligation of contribution; the kind, character, and number of disagreements the team has over issues and what processes are used to resolve them; the use of information resources, both information available and how information is managed by the team; how the team members relate, work, and interact with each other; how often the team meets; the issues that get dealt with; the issues that are unresolved; and finally the human dynamic issues. Of importance are those issues which relate to interpersonal communication, styles, competition, interaction, relatedness, and trust. All of these are challenges that will be confronted on the way to building team effectiveness. There are techniques and processes identified in this book that help the team members get past any barriers or challenges they might confront. The issue is using them and making the requisite of team functionality the basic underpinning for successful work and achievement of outcomes of the team.

Phase III: Team Working

Each of these phases depends on success achieved in the previous phase. Clearly, an effective, operating, functional team requires that the formation of purpose and direction and the resolution of process, issues, and challenges are required for the functional appropriateness of team process. Most of the activities of building good team process will be related to the kind and character of the relationships the team members have with each other and how consistently they operate: first, to make the team effective, and second, to achieve the team's outcomes. Good working relationships within the context of the team are critical.

Peer relationships

Productive processes require certain components to be in place for teams to be effective. The following are critical elements to organize the team's effectiveness as the team is underway in deliberating its issues.

BOX **3-8**

Initial Challenges With Teams

- Personal agendas
- Group conflict
- Communication styles
- Roles
- Personal relationships
- Variable contributions
- Level of skill
- Group expectations
- Good information

Mentorship and good facilitation are critical at the outset of team formation. Through this process, the rougher developmental stages can be better handled and conflicts can be confronted early in the process. Trust of the facilitator is critical to team building.

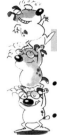

People quickly lose interest in activities that have no results and do not make a difference. Methodology helps prevent this from happening.

A. Establish an agenda. An agenda, either formal or informal, helps discipline the process of teamwork and team deliberation (Team Tip 3-3). Every member of the team should be working toward some common goal or some common achievement; therefore when the group gathers or when the group informally meets there should be some expectation that it is essentially fulfilling the requirements of an agenda to which all members agree. The agenda should relate specifically to a goal around which the team has been constructed, and as it undertakes issues related to those goals, the agenda should reflect progress against what it is expected to accomplish. Either formally in group meetings or informally in work processes, the group should always be unfolding its activities within the context of its purpose and objectives. Therefore agenda in this case relates more to a common understanding each member of the team has with regard to the team purpose imbedded in any one of the functions and activities it has related to its goals.

B. A common understanding. All members of the team should be clear about their relationship to the purposes, objectives, functions, and activities expected of the team. Certainly, the team wants to be able to fulfill its requirements. To do so means being sure that all members are certain about not only their own contribution, but the contribution of others. Clarity around that relationship will eliminate much ambiguity and foundation for conflict. Because conflict needs to be avoided wherever possible or confronted whenever necessary, the team wants to make sure that it is clear regarding expectations around both roles and functions.

C. Team meeting methodology. Each team should have a methodology for effectively undertaking its work and managing its meeting times. A formalized and consistent method for conducting the meeting is critical to its success. Using tools and format to keep a meeting on target and producing outcomes is essential to maintaining team member interest. Because clinical teams have special constraints around the issues of time and work assignment, any meetings that are scheduled must be efficient, effective, brief, and successful. Clinical providers do not have as much option to access each other as frequently as other kinds of teams might have. Therefore each time a team meets formally it should be an efficient and effective exercise that can be done with a great deal of participation, satisfaction, and achievement of outcomes. All the models of progress around teams should clearly have processes in place where the goals of the meeting and team interaction are clear; where the team is able to deal with its issues with effective methodology; where meaningful, viable, and immediately effective process is undertaken; where mechanisms and methodologies around data collection and analysis are undertaken; where specific and appropriate action, both individual and collective responses, can be clearly outlined; and where an appropriate closure and follow-up process is identified. Each of these process items is essential to the effectiveness of any team gathering to meet formally or informally to undertake its work. From goals, to team relationship, to process effectiveness, to data processes, to action steps, to closure and follow-up, each team member must play a role in fulfilling the requirements of good team process. Each of the elements identified is essential to continuous and effective processing of any team at any level.

This chapter has focused specifically on basic and initial activities of team formation in the first three phases of team development. Introduced are the fundamental processes associated with ensuring that the team can become functional. Addressing each of the issues of team formation becomes essential to the sustainability of the team and the team members' ability to work well together and achieve the team's purposes. In the next chapter we will continue to focus on team development with an emphasis on creating effective and well-functioning teams.

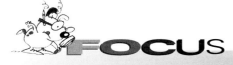

FOCUS

Required Team Attributes

- Purpose
- Goals
- Methodology
- Accountability
- Clear Roles
- Trust
- Good facilitation
- Outcomes

Bibliography

Adams F, Hansen G: *Putting democracy to work,* San Francisco, Berrett-Koehler Publishers, 1993.

Barker J: Tightening the iron cage: concertive control in self managed teams, *Administrative Science Quarterly* 38(3):408-437, 1993.

Fisher K: *Leading self-directed work teams,* New York, McGraw-Hill, Inc, 1995.

Graham M, Lebaron M: *The horizontal revolution: guiding the teaming takeover,* San Francisco, Jossey-Bass, 1994.

Katzenbach J, Smith D: *The wisdom of teams,* Boston, McKinsey & Company, 1993.

Kottler J: *Beyond blame: a new way of resolving conflicts in relationship,* San Francisco, Jossey-Bass, 1996.

Lipman-Blumen J: *The connective edge: leading in an interdependent world,* San Francisco, Jossey-Bass, 1996.

Maurer G: True empowerment: from shared governance to self managed work teams, *Journal of Shared Governance* 1(1):25-30, 1995.

Mohrman S, Cohen S, Mohrman A: *Designing team based organizations,* San Francisco, Jossey-Bass, 1995.

Myers K: Games companies play and how to stop them, *Training* June, 68-70, 1992.

Pacanowsky M: Team tools for wicked problems, *Organizational Dynamics* 23(2):36-51, 1995.

Parker G: *Cross functional teams,* San Francisco, Jossey-Bass, 1994.

Pedersen A, Easton L: Teamwork: bringing order out of chaos, *Nursing Management* 26(6):34-35, 1995.

Schutz W: *The human element: workers and the bottom line,* San Francisco, Jossey-Bass, 1994.

Shipper F, Manz C: Employee self-management without formally designated teams: an alternative road to empowerment, *Organizational Dynamics* 20(3):48-63, 1992.

Ulschak F, SnowAntle S: *Team architecture: the manager's guide to building effective work teams,* Chicago, Health Administration Press, 1995.

Watkins K, Marsick V: *Sculpting the learning organization,* San Francisco, Jossey-Bass, 1993.

Wellins R, Byham W, Wilson J: *Empowered teams,* San Francisco, Jossey-Bass, 1993.

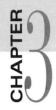

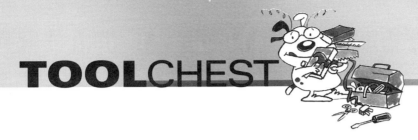TOOLCHEST

TOOLA: Team Empowerment Exercise

Purpose of the Exercise

This exercise is to help team members identify what they can do to become more effective and more aware of teamwork and the ability to make decisions together. This exercise focuses on the ability of the team to act in an empowered way.

Team Size

The group should not exceed more than ten members.

Time Required

About 2 hours.

Place

This exercise should be undertaken in a room large enough to allow the team to be comfortable and to use a flip chart. Usually working at a round table is helpful to the team process.

Supplies

An easel, a large blackboard, a flip chart, markers, and masking tape are useful for this exercise.

Instruction and Activity

The team leader outlines the principles of empowerment and the application of that empowerment in the process of decision making and team rela-

tionship building. Using these concepts and a facilitator provides the foundation for understanding the principles of empowerment in making the team more effective.

The team leader then asks the team members to build a list of methods and mechanisms that they suggest will facilitate their involvement in decision making and in solution seeking. Following that, the team members clarify and outline the list of elements that will, they believe, make the team more empowered and more successful. The team members select the five highest-priority items or actions that they think represent the most empowered processes. After having selected these items, the team members identify specific ways in which their priorities can be implemented within the context of the team process.

Following the identification of the priorities and the action steps related to it, the team facilitator identifies with the group ways in which team members can incorporate their recommendations into the group process. The team leader then summarizes their recommendations, indicates how they will next be used, and sets the time frame for the next team meeting in which these processes will be applied.

At the next meeting the recommendations of the team group are applied, and following the meeting an evaluation of their application is undertaken by the team and the team leader in about a 15-minute activity.

TOOL B: Day-To-Day, Self-Managed Team Process

In *Business Without Bosses,** C. C. Manns and H. P. Simms identify that there are many functional and routine things that a team must do to undertake its work. Each of these activities is related to the day-to-day functional processes associated with self-managed work teams. Building self-managed work teams in a way that is effective and meaningful is a critical part of moving teams into sustainability. Each of these elements is identified as a checkoff for the ongoing functional and productive activities of making teams workable.

Instructions: This checkoff list contains the following elements that each team leader will need to incorporate into the processes associated with day-to-day team experiences.

Team responsibilities and day-to-day activities:
- ❑ Select team members.
- ❑ Identify team leaders.
- ❑ Ensure that specific role assignments and work group obligations are identified.
- ❑ Enumerate new membership training and orientation process.
- ❑ Determine and outline the rules of engagement.
- ❑ Determine work process and team-based relationships.
- ❑ Establish schedules and assignments around team process.

* Manns CC, Simms HP: *Business without bosses*, New York, John Wiley & Sons, 1993.

- ❑ Make specific role assignments within the work group or team.
- ❑ Determine appropriate support material or work material necessary to do the work of the team.
- ❑ Establish a process for record keeping and work group process.
- ❑ Determine the quality control, measurement, and improvement data process.
- ❑ Outline specific needs for materials, processes, and information.
- ❑ Select and dismiss members as indicated through the rules of engagement.
- ❑ Establish times for the regular, at least weekly, group meetings.
- ❑ Establish the accountability framework for the group.
- ❑ Define consequences of performance and nonperformance.
- ❑ Outline the disciplines for specific, unacceptable behavior.
- ❑ Identify the characteristics and functions around performance, feedback, and team evaluation processes.
- ❑ Identify the communication, generation, and information sharing process.

Self-managed work teams are unique in their own composition; however, they have elements within them that are characteristic of all teams. The above items are a part of the content of almost any team, but they have specific importance within the context of self-managed teams. Increasingly, as teams develop they need to control and monitor their own processes, functions, and activities, as well as undertake appropriate evaluation of their work. Using the above developmental and day-to-day process items helps keep a team focused on the functional components that must be in place at all times to ensure the team's effectiveness.

TOOL C: Getting Started with Teams

Organizational Issues and Notes

Organizational change is frequently traumatic, noisy, and stressful for organizations and individuals. Such processes are seldom as easy as they appear to be. Each individual must be aware of and sensitive to the impact the change will have on each component of the organization and other persons in the system.

Instructions: Following are items that need to be assessed by the individuals as they begin to confront the issues of change and their role in relationship to it. Identifying some of these realities becomes critical to having a reality orientation in the face of change.

- Things are the way they are, and that is where you begin.
  - ❑ Can you accept your organization where it is now?
  - ❑ Can you see the need for change emerge within the organization?
  - ❑ Has the organization been stable or quiet for a long period of time?
- Nothing remains the same.
  - ❑ How do you feel about change?
  - ❑ Does change stress you?
  - ❑ Are you good at initiating changes when the need arises?
- It takes a lot of people to make change.
  - ❑ What is the general attitude toward change in your part of the organization?
  - ❑ Do you have co-workers who find change difficult?
  - ❑ Is your unit or department adverse to the issues surrounding change?
- Resistance is normal.
  - ❑ Can you identify how your resistance is manifested?
  - ❑ Can you name any specific events where your resistance was clear?
  - ❑ How will you deal with your natural resistance to change as you confront it?

The above questions relate specifically to accommodation for change and getting started with moving toward a different format for the organization. Teams require the individual to begin to dialogue with others about personal issues and relational processes. All teams require some level of clarity and honesty in individuals before they confront building relationships with others. Answering these questions and reflecting on what they imply will provide a foundation for deliberating on the issues affecting the development of teams.

TOOL D: Identified Losses and Gains Survey

In the midst of change all of us move from what we know into areas of concern, confusion, uncertainty, or fear. Imbedded in all these changes are many losses that express or enumerate the comfort, satisfaction, confidence, and competence of our own work or practice. Identifying loss and being able to deal with it directly is a critical element of the ability to embrace and engage change. Enumerating losses becomes critical to our ability to understand what the change means to us and to be able to undertake the activities necessary to imbed the changes in our own lives.

Group Size: No More Than Ten Individuals

Instructions for the Group Exercise

The facilitator gathers the group and identifies the purpose of the gathering. The facilitator enumerates issues of change and the struggles and problems associated with initiating change and personal adaptation to it. With this introduction the facilitator leads the group to the process of identifying losses.

After the facilitator has identified the specific loss events, situations, or occurrences, each individual is instructed to identify on a clean sheet of paper what she or he will most miss or feel about the change that is occurring. Each person is asked to identify the loss in specific terms as it has meaning for that person individually in his or her own life experience. The identification should be as specific, as concrete, and as clear as possible.

The facilitator then moves around the room encouraging each person to share his or her personal experience of loss. Also encouraged should be whatever personal response or feelings are attached to the sense of loss the individual expresses. Each individual should be permitted sufficient time to express in personal terms the meaning of his or her loss in a way that best meets individual needs.

Following the completion of the expression of losses around the room, the facilitator encourages all participants to take their sheet of paper and place it in a box, a bowl, or other container in the room. Some groups may even want to put it in a container with a door or a lid that can close on all of the sheets containing the enumerated losses. Once these sheets have been deposited the facilitator draws the group around the container, joins hands with the group, and concludes the exercise with the understanding that now that the losses have been expressed, they have been shared and communicated, and now have been placed in the container. As the participants leave the room they must leave their losses in the container as they go forth to embrace and engage the changes they must confront. Through this exercise the individual concerns, issues, fears, and doubts related to the loss of current activities, confidence, competence, or other indicators can be expressed and people can move on to address needed changes.

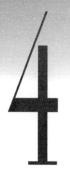

Getting Started: Making Teams Work

Ours is a brand new world. Time has ceased, space has vanished. We now live in a global village.

Marshall McLuhan

The first three phases of team formation are essentially developmental. They are filled with activities that provide a functional and relational foundation for good team functioning. The subsequent activities of team formation require that these foundations be in place before the team can mature and keep its focus on its work and outcomes instead of the team's formation and relationship issues. Ensuring that members are capable of functioning and relating is the beginning point for a renewed focus on the work and products of the team's efforts. This is the essential role of evaluation, feedback, and conflict resolution.

EVALUATE BEHAVIOR AND PERFORMANCE OF TEAM MEMBERS

In the team-building process, the relationships and interactions among members are critical to the team's success. No team can be sustained for long without addressing the behavioral expectations, roles, and relationships of all members. The greatest problems in almost all team-based organizations are the conflicts that are generated out of problems associated with relationships and interactions. Clinical teams are no different from any other kind of team. These behaviors and interactions are continually

Team behavior is the foundation for building relationships. Sustainable teams can address their members' issues and relationships as an ongoing part of doing the work.

influenced by the ebb and flow of the work and relationships of each team member. Of greatest concern on most clinical teams is the role of the physician among other providers. Physicians have historically been most loosely associated with the health care team. They essentially have been the "guests" of the system, bringing patients, documenting activities, and essentially leaving to complete roles and obligations within the contexts of their own individual practices. With team-based approaches, there is a demand for a more integrated and a more intensive activity between team members and the physician. Indeed the physician is considered as an active member of the team (Box 4-1).

Much of the initial work of team building along the critical paths and within the context of integrated, interdisciplinary teams will be around involving the physician and other team members and observing, evaluating, and addressing behavioral, relational, and interactional problems associated with working between and among the variety of disciplines, including the physician, within the context of the team. There must be substantive evidence at all levels of the team that the team is committed to the same goals, relationships, and interactions with each other, and that commitment results in meaningful outcomes as well as sustenance for the team itself. Effective team building involves digesting and clarifying issues around the basic relationship of team members with each other.

CREATING MEANINGFUL FEEDBACK LOOPS

Much of the relationship involved in any team framework relates to the generation, management, and communication of information. Work-based teams require accurate, meaningful, and viable information as the foundation for their work. Communication of information is one of the more critical aspects of effective team processing. Timely communication, feedback, and response are critical to the ongoing success of the team. Therefore feedback mechanisms that are prompt, accurate, immediate, and provide what is needed by both teams and the individual members are essential to building effective trust on the team and to sustaining the team's work.

BOX 4-1

Cues for Including Physicians

- Schedule the times of meetings for times the doctor can be there.
- Make sure there is a reason for the physician to be there.
- Help the physician feel comfortable in deliberating with other team members.
- Resolve personal difficulties between members early in the team-building process.
- Focus on patient and clinical concerns; physicians are interested in the care patients receive.
- Use the clinical protocols, best practices, or care maps as the centerpiece for dialogue and the foundation for building communication.
- Deal with communication problems as soon as they arise.

It is not the role of the manager to be translator in team-based approaches; the manager facilitates the development of effective communication skills in all the staff.

Without accurate and meaningful information generated in a timely way, and without good feedback mechanisms, the team has nothing to sustain it (Box 4-2). Information is the life blood of teamwork and therefore communication between members; the generation of information to all members becomes a critical part of the process of ensuring the effectiveness of a team. The team simply cannot wait to do its fundamental work; therefore it needs whatever tools are essential to that work and will require that those tools be generated freely and openly. Team performance is based on ensuring that appropriate team communication processes are in place.

COLLABORATION AND CONFLICT

As mentioned earlier, relationship building is fundamental to the sustenance of any team. Teams collaborate at varying levels and have varying levels of conflict. Teams move continuously through cycles of collaboration and cycles of conflict. Often these two cycles may be operating at the same time. It should be anticipated that both conflict and collaboration will occur at the same time and within the context of the team. You cannot bring individuals together with varying backgrounds, insights, and roles without generating some level of conflict. Conflict is normative in diverse work groups; it is to be anticipated and expected. For teams to be successful it must even be embraced. Team leadership must develop processes appropriate to dealing with conflict and ensuring that it gets addressed appropriately (Box 4-3).

Collaboration and conflict are two sides of the same coin. Collaborative activities must also be continually addressed and embraced as a part of the work of the team. Collaboration requires that all team members be interested in what the other members have to contribute to the team's work. They have to be open and responsive to the ideas and notions of others around the work. They have to be able to incorporate new ideas in their own practice that come from other team members, as well as generate new ideas for others (Box 4-4). Collaboration also indicates respect for others in terms of their differences both in approach and in action.

BOX **4-2**

Feedback
• Is clear
• Is direct
• Is understood
• Is timely
• Is accurate

BOX **4-3**

Conflict Resolution Process
• Identify the circumstances.
• Look for a central theme.
• Identify the issue.
• Locate accountability.
• Assign accountability.
• Enumerate solution methods.
• Apply or implement suggested approaches.
• Regather to evaluate progress.
• Apply strategies again.

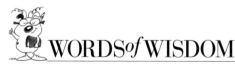

WORDS*of*WISDOM

Nothing is worse than not getting feedback about work or performance. Information is the life blood of good relationships; it is critical to share it generously.

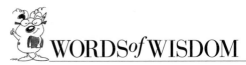

WORDS of WISDOM

Conflict is normal and should be anticipated in team formation and management. What is important is that it be handled well!

~

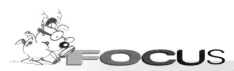

FOCUS

Barriers to Collaboration

Many elements of a relationship can create barriers to collaboration that require a process of resolution. Issues that can create barriers include the following:

- *An inability to put the real issues on the table*
- *Personal dishonesty in one or several of the members of the team*
- *No real method or process for making it safe to deal with the issues impeding relationships*
- *Uncertainty around role and relationship between members of the team*
- *Absence of team members at the time committed to problem resolution*
- *No real team commitment or identity*
- *No accountability or performance expectation that makes a difference*

One of the most difficult arenas in clinical teams is recognizing that a whole range of actions can achieve the same outcomes without requiring rote or standardized action. Approaches to rendering appropriate clinical services are often different. People use different techniques and processes depending on the individual's background, experience, and skills. If the principles are adhered to and if appropriate outcomes are achieved through a tightness of fit between process and those outcomes, the differences and approaches should be respected by each of the individual team members. Teamwork grows through the openness of all members to the opportunity to learn, broaden, and incorporate new practices into a member's own work. This openness and availability will enhance the creativity, strength, viability, and sustenance of effective teamwork.

MAKING DECISIONS

Much goes into making effective decisions. Decisions are not simply effective because groups make them. Good decisions require discipline, methodology, and an effective, replicable process that continually bears

BOX 4-4

Requisites for Collaboration

Collaboration is a skill set, not a gift. It can be learned, but not without a process that involves all team members. A good process is necessary. Requisites for collaboration are:

- Learning process around the principles
- Situations of collaboration enumerated
- Barriers to collaboration enumerated
- Expectations for performance clarified
- Action learning and practice processes undertaken
- Problem areas focused on and worked out
- Method of issue confrontation and resolution applied
- Regular time for evaluating progress and need for skill

positive results (Box 4-5). In team-based processing specific individuals do not make all the decisions for the team. If there is a team leadership position it is not the expectation of the team leader to make decisions for the team, but instead to facilitate the team's decision-making process. Therefore effective methodology and good critical decision skills are essential components of all of the team members' functioning in relation to their own work and in interaction with the team. Using the techniques identified in other sections of this book for decision making and for ensuring effective team processing will be critical to the sustenance of the team. Decision making is a critical centerpiece of the work of teams. Therefore careful and studied attention should be paid to the methods and techniques used for creating effective decisions in the organization.

FINAL PHASE: SYNERGISTIC TEAMS

The final stage of goal attainment for building effective teams is synergistic team performance. Synergistic teams function continuously and regularly at a high level of function, achieve outcomes regularly, and operate in a manner that is satisfactory to team members and to the organization. Peak-performing teams have methods and mechanisms for addressing their issues and concerns in effective and meaningful ways. Peak-performing teams have mechanisms in place for continuing their motivation and ensuring the appropriateness of their actions, activities, and relationships with each other and the organization, as well as other teams in the system.

Staying Motivated

Maintaining the motivation of the team as it works to operate as the modus operandi of the organization is critical to good functioning. This requires a continuous encouragement of participation and ownership, investment, and involvement of all of the members. It requires the leader to continually reenergize and reengage the players in the process of deliberation in building their relationships with each other. Obviously, reactivating and reinitiating team processes, changing the dynamics of team interaction and

---

BOX **4-5**

Essentials of Decision Making
• Good decision methods
• Solid information
• Good support system
• Critical thinking skills
• Good evaluation processes
• Validation of learning/application
• Good error assessment
• Effective corrective action process
• Effective collective deliberations
• Meaningful feedback loops
• Good management support structure

Synergy is achieved when the parts, components, or people are working together such that the sum of their actions together is greater than the combined force of their actions separately.

Motivation is not the responsibility of the manager: it is the obligation of each individual. The leader simply provides the opportunity to converge the changes in the organization with the mindset of the team. Each person is responsible for the work of clarifying and committing to the changes that affect his or her life.

Staying centered on the purposes and objectives of the team's work is central to the team's ability to thrive and grow. Nothing is worse than losing sight of the purpose of the team and getting lost in the process. When that happens the whole world of the team becomes the latest events and processes, and meaning disappears. It is the obligation of team leadership to continuously validate the team's understanding and work around the purposes that give it meaning.

TEAM**TIP**   4.1

Celebrate Success

Success should be celebrated. The small, incremental successes define the strength of a team. Every team should take a moment in its process and work to celebrate the successes that enumerate the team's value and contribution to the patient and the system. Failing to acclaim the successes achieved along the way leads to failure to recognize real contribution and ultimately affects the creativity, enthusiasm, and motivation of every team member.

method, and continually challenging the team to higher levels of performance are the requisites of leadership as a team reaches peak levels of performance. Leadership will require continual renewal and advancement in terms of learning about techniques and processes that engage the team and challenge it to further and growing levels of development and improvement. This requires leaders to remain one step ahead of the challenges and circumstances that can diminish the team's enthusiasm or slowly destroy the team's effectiveness.

Staying On Track

Keeping the team on track in terms of its purpose, mission, goals, objectives, and direction will also be an important part of the team process. Leadership will have to continue not only to stimulate the team, but to evaluate the team with regard to performance and outcome. Certainly, outcome will determine the effectiveness and value of the team and its work. Validating the processes and practices of the team against the outcomes anticipated and achieved becomes a critical evaluative process that determines just how effective and valid the team process has been. That method will continually be a part of the team's obligation to its own commitment. Satisfactorily achieving its goals should also be a source of renewal and heightened interest in advancing its work.

Celebrating Success

Finally, it is important for the team to celebrate successes as it advances (Team Tip 4-1). The successes that it looks at should be celebrated from the very inception of the team process. From small successes to the great successes of team accomplishment and outcome achievement, each member of the team should be able to enumerate his or her contribution to the successful development of the team process. One of the greatest problems with team enthusiasm and commitment over the long term is the fact that team celebrations are not undertaken within the context of work. Therefore work eventually becomes looked at as tedious and routine, rote and uninspiring.

Celebrating and joining with each other in moments of acknowledgment of accomplishment, growth, change, and advancement becomes a way of stimulating and developing the strong relationships of the team and its commitment to its ongoing success. Developing personal relationships and building the dynamic of that relationship can only be enhanced through the process of encouraging periodic and frequent celebrations of success.

Each of the four steps of team building is critical to the initial phases of developing team growth. The foundations that are established for team effectiveness become the critical base on which the team will grow. If flaws or failures, inadequacy or inability to address the key fundamental issues are not taken care of in the initial stages of team development, they will come to haunt the success and effectiveness of the team in later stages.

Team leadership must be aware of the necessity for establishing firm underpinnings for the unfolding activities of the team. In the process of undertaking teamwork there will be ample opportunities for challenge, conflict, uncertainty, and further refinement and development of the team. That can be expected as the ongoing dynamic associated with developing and maintaining team processes. Attending to the basic four steps that undergird the development of teams can ensure a strong foundation on which subsequent teamwork can advance and improve both the actions and outcomes of the team and the organization.

THE UNIQUE CHARACTER OF INTERDISCIPLINARY TEAMS

In health care the focus on interdisciplinary activities is becoming an increasingly important part of structuring team-based work. Many organizations have broken down the departmental, compartmentalized, vertically defined structures of the organization in an effort to build more collaborative, cohesive, and integrated approaches to delivering patient care services. While some of these initial efforts have been successful, others have not. Defining the functions, activities, roles, relationships, expectations, and outcomes of these processes is an impor-

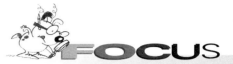

Small Successes

- *Good decision*
- *Conflict resolved*
- *Problem solved*
- *Patient satisfied*
- *Good team meeting*
- *Small cost savings*
- *New approaches worked well*
- *New procedure mastered*
- *Satisfaction survey improved*
- *Personal or team achievement obtained*
- *New learning, good results*
- *JCAHO likes what the team is doing*
- *Budget approved as submitted*
- *Degree/certification completed*
- *Doctors are happy*
- *Staff members are happy*
- *Another year of challenges well met*

Interdisciplinary better describes teams than multidisciplinary. It enumerates the character of relationship that is necessary to build effective teams. The unique character of teams reflects a strong emphasis on interaction between the members and the disciplines they represent.

BOX 4-6

Stages of Interdisciplinary Team Construction

- Each discipline is clear about its practice foundations and parameters.
- All team members bring to the table their expectations and perceptions of their work and contribution.
- The terms of engagement for the team are identified at the outset so that expectations are clear.
- The identity and framework of the team are articulated early to generate a new identity for the members.
- The work of the team is outlined regarding its members, relationship, and expectations for performance.
- Position descriptions, accountability, and role relationships are worked out among the members.
- The team implements, evaluates, and adjusts its role as it implements the team format in clinical service.

Interdisciplinary team formation has the same processes associated with it as any other team format, but it demands a commitment of the disciplines to join together in a common effort and agreement around the patient to ensure that all provider activity acts in concert in the patient's best interest.

tant first step in ensuring that there is a sustained and abiding growth in team-based approaches to delivering patient care. The challenges in doing so are many. It can be expected in every organization developing interdisciplinary teams that many of the aspects and characteristics of such teams will challenge the very foundations of the design and structuring of hospitals and health systems in fundamental and meaningful ways (Box 4-6). To build sustainable and valuable team processes resulting in meaningful clinical outcomes, much of what is currently in place will have to be challenged, adapted, and changed in many critical and fundamental ways.

Interdisciplinary teams cannot be sustained unless there is a critical balance between the character of individual members and the expectations of team performance. Much of the conflict in developing interdisciplinary teams arises in this arena of individual accountability versus the accountability of the team. It has not always been clear what the accountabilities of individual roles are, let alone what the aggregated accountability of the team is. The interdisciplinary team takes its focus and its foundation in clarifying the roles between individual team members and the collective accountability in the obligation of the team.

No one approach or formula can guarantee interdisciplinary team success. The culture of the organization, the focus of patient care, the character of the interdisciplinary interactions, and the purposes and roles of the team will all have an influence on the kind and character of interdisciplinary team development.

BUILDING ON FIRM FOUNDATIONS

The foundations of interdisciplinary teams should reflect the foundation for any team development. Many of the approaches covered in the first part of this chapter and subsequent chapters on team function, development, and efficiency also form the foundations of any approach to interdisciplinary activities. These firm foundations are critical to the establishment of effective relationship building in an interdisciplinary framework. Therefore the following key elements will be essential to the firm foundations for any clinical team:

1. Structure of the team
2. Communication and interaction among team members
3. Effective team design
4. Clarification of accountability
5. Relationship building
6. Process activities
7. Terms of reference
8. Outcome-based evaluation

Each of the above requires specific activities to ensure that the underpinnings of the interdisciplinary approach are firm and can provide a framework within which specific interdisciplinary processes can unfold.

GOOD COMMUNICATION STRATEGIES

In interdisciplinary team building the communication between team members becomes critical (Team Tip 4-2). Each of the disciplines brings with it a frame of reference that is unique to its discipline. Therefore the language, thought processes, focus, and elements of practice are unique to each discipline. As team members come together around the same table they bring all of those precepts with them, requiring the formation of a common foundation, a common language, and a method of integration that will be necessary to sustain their relationship. Therefore communication technique and methodology will be critical to the success of the processes of developing interdisciplinary approaches (Box 4-7). Valuing each of the members and ensuring that everyone contributes to the team's success, and incorporating the language, culture, customs, and issues into the dialogue of seeking common ground, will be important parts of the interdisciplinary process.

Recognizing the differences that each team member brings is as important as trying to find the common elements. Specific and unique accountability and contribution will be based on these differences. It is expected

TEAMTIP   4.2

Team Meeting Tool

Good communication strategies begin with the use of a format or tools for communication. One essential tool for team-based interaction is the use of a flip chart. No team meetings should ever occur without the use of a flip chart. This tool helps clarify all processes and can evidence whether the work is leading to any outcome.

BOX 4-7

Group Communication Steps
1. Clarify the reason everyone is gathered.
2. Outline the time frame for the meeting.
3. Identify the agenda.
4. Define a method for addressing each issue.
5. Select techniques for full group participation.
6. Use a flip chart for process work.
7. Validate understanding and progress of work.
8. Restate decisions.
9. Certify that agreement has been reached.
10. Define follow-up activities, next meeting, and agenda.

BOX 4-8

Measuring Team Performance

- Determine a standard of performance.
- Define measurement criteria.
- Create a measurement tool.
- Fit the tool with the group's work processes.
- Define increments of measure.
- Ensure group understanding and acceptance of measurement process.
- Outline individual and group competence requirements.
- Enumerate consequences of normative and unacceptable performance in advance.
- Define mechanisms and processes for measurement and review.
- Evaluate, affirm, and undertake corrective action.

that these differences will be maintained. Unlike other teams, where there is a stronger integration of consciousness into the team framework, the unique disciplines contributing to the interdisciplinary team will have to be maintained throughout the team's process, and these contributions will have to continually be identified as unique and appropriate within the context of the disciplines' contributions.

Team performance should continuously be measured. Measurement of performance evidences clarity of understanding of its contribution to the outcomes of work (Box 4-8). Therefore clearly defined, discipline-specific, and integrated performance measurement processes must be incorporated into interdisciplinary teams. The performance evaluation processes require a 360-degree orientation so that performance measurement both inside and outside the discipline can be undertaken consistent with the expectations of the team. Therefore the team must have team-based evaluative processes, discipline-specific evaluative criteria, and organizational evaluation mechanisms that measure the team's performance against the objectives or outcomes to which it is directed. There are three levels of team evaluation: individual, coactive team, and outcome. These three characteristics are the critical elements of ensuring effective and viable performance within the context of the team in an interdisciplinary frame of reference

BOX 4-9

Three Levels of Team Evaluation

Individual. Performance of team members is the focus of this team-based and team-driven evaluation process.

Coactive team. The team is the focus of this evaluation and includes all members of the team evaluating the collective effectiveness of the activities and relationship of team members.

Outcome. This is the evaluation process combining the team and the system's review of the results of team activities and their "fit" with the goals and expectation for the team's work.

(Box 4-9). Performance measurements therefore will require a focus on outcomes, an ability to see the whole instead of parts so that the overall impact or effect of work is clearly identified. An indication of investment, ownership, and commitment to the process from the point-of-service throughout the organization and a depth of understanding of the contribution of each member of the team to the critical paths and to the outcomes are basic team requisites. Focus on outcomes, an ability to see the whole, investment in ownership, and a depth of understanding of the contribution to outcomes form the critical framework for the evaluative process in interdisciplinary teams.

ESTABLISHING THE DISCIPLINARY PARAMETERS

In interdisciplinary teams the parameters of each of the disciplines must not only be respected but clearly articulated. Each discipline brings with it a knowledge base, professional identification, service roles and activities, and a set of expectations unique to that discipline. These elements form the foundation for the parameters of that discipline. They must be as clear to team members as the interaction and integration activities of the team. The disciplines bring with them specific and clearly enumerated accountabilities that are a part of both their social mandate and their functional role. These mandates identify the discipline in a unique way that requires the discipline to be respected and honored in terms of the contribution that it brings.

Contrary to much of what is believed about interdisciplinary teams, it is not the intent of integration and team-based activities to diminish the impact, the role, or the value of any given discipline. Indeed, it is to advance that discipline and to ensure that it is incorporated consistently within the expectations of team performance and the measurement of team outcomes. The price the organization pays for this is less delineation of the team's functions and roles within a compartmentalized, departmental structure and more linkage around the point-of-service driven from the patient care culture into the organization rather than from the provider toward the pa-

Elimination of the unique contribution of the professions should never be a part of redesign or team formation. Teams respect the diversity of contribution that comes from their members with different perspectives and roles to play as team members. The integration of the unique contributions of each member brings meaning to the team and value to its accomplishments.

TEAM PROCESS REQUIREMENTS

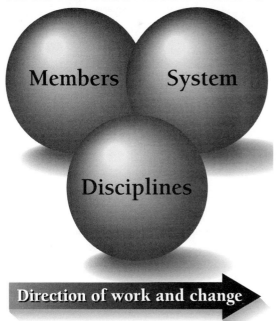

TEAM INTEGRATION

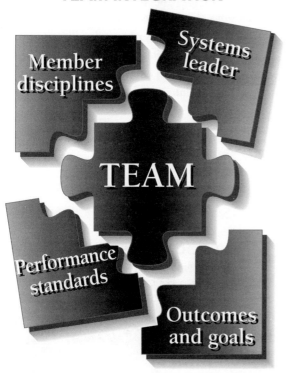

The culture of the service defines the membership and diversity of the team. Each clinical setting will have its own configuration of service. This will require that the teams that are formed be unique to the needs of that service. Teams should never be consistently defined across the system. To do so defeats the purpose of team-based design.

tient. This means in essence that the disciplines begin to define themselves within the context of their mutual and unique contribution to patient outcomes rather than to clinical process.

Using patient outcomes and their impact on those outcomes as the anchor to their function or relationships, each discipline begins to identify itself more clearly in relationship to the other disciplines with which it associates. When it does so, each discipline begins to see itself in terms of its contribution to patient outcomes and its role in relationship to others who also contribute to those same outcomes in a differentiated way. Differentiated roles becomes the defining heart of the interdisciplinary team-based approach.

The challenge of these approaches is evidenced in the focus each discipline has on its function and activities. When it begins to focus on outcomes and the processes that it facilitates, each discipline begins to see that there can be a shift in functions and activities and the locus of control for many of those functions traditionally assumed to operate under the auspices of any one given discipline. Here is where cross-training, integration, multifocal service, and shared accountabilities begin to become more clearly defined.

As the disciplines mature in dialogue and within the context of team, they start moving away from functional, task-oriented delineations of work to more outcome orientations and relational understandings of the impact each discipline has on the team's outcome. In this way the focus from task and function shifts toward accountability and outcome. The shift in this focus provides a stronger basis on which to more clearly articulate the disciplines' relationships with each other, rather than simply the differences that each discipline bring to the relationship.

INTERDISCIPLINARY LEADERSHIP

One of the unique concerns of the interdisciplinary team is the need for good leadership. Often much of the leadership of interdisciplinary teams is provided by nurses and nursing. This is not because nurses are specifically gifted in leadership out of context of the role of other disciplines and their ability to lead. It is primarily because of the character of the nurse's role in coordinating, integrating, and facilitating the continuum of care. Nurses have historically been educated, prepared, and experienced in integrating and coordinating a broad base of services in the patient's ongoing journey through the institutional system. This coordinative and integrative function, and the activities associated with it, has been a fundamental part of the nursing expectation since the initiation of hospital-based practice. As a result, much of the role of the nurse is amenable to interdisciplinary team leadership. However, this need not always be the case.

Depending on the culture, function, and priorities of a particular practice environment, critical path, or continuum of care, different practitioners may have the obligation to provide leadership within particular pathways. These patient pathways serve as the foundation for determining the appropriate leadership for teams within the context of that culture. Leadership therefore becomes less a discipline-specific expectation and more a patient pathway expectation.

Each patient in the system has a particular set of needs at any given time that are exemplified in the patient's relationship to the health pathway. In that framework there is an expectation that the pathway would determine the activities, functions, and expectations for that patient in that given set of circumstances. Certain pathways, such as women's health, rehabilitation, and mental health services, may attend to a variety of disciplines depending on the need, the point-of-service, and the particular culture of service a patient requires at any given point in the patient's relationship with the system. Therefore leadership is determined based on need, not based on discipline.

The discipline providing leadership is further determined by the culture within which the service is provided and the needs that culture represents to the patient served. Therefore leadership is a subset of the patient's environment, not a requisite of the provider's role. However, that need and that culture determine the character of the leader and who should provide leadership in any given set of circumstances.

THREE ELEMENTS OF TEAM SUSTAINABILITY

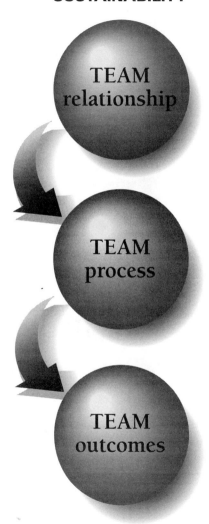

TEAM relationship

TEAM process

TEAM outcomes

TEAM FOCUS

Right members

Right process

Good evaluation

Patient

Right outcome

WORDS*of* WISDOM

The key to effective and sustainable teams is leadership. It does not matter what kind of configuration an organization has: the leadership of the team is critical to its success. No team fails by neglect alone—it is usually actively led into its own demise.

A great deal of dialogue and discussion remains around team leadership, case management, and other newly emerging roles within the health care system. Each of the discussions has imbedded in it issues around role, leadership, and control. Although it is important to incorporate each of these elements in the dialogue, it is equally important to make sure that leadership is provided based on the needs of those served and the framework and design of the system supporting how that service unfolds.

The emerging roles of leadership around mentorship, outcome orientation, innovation, interdisciplinary relationship, point-of-service design, and team-based approaches all change the very character and content of leadership roles. Each of these must be considered in both management and team leadership roles, how those roles are defined, and who is assigned to provide them.

INTERTEAM ISSUES

As organizations build more continua of care and integrated interdisciplinary organizational systems, there will be more opportunities for team relationships across the system (Team Tip 4-3). The challenges associated with this will be considerable. Since most organizations have been operating in departmental, silo-based structures for generations, most workers in those systems have grown up in just such structures. Trying to learn to work as an integrated whole, visioning one's role within the context of the whole, and looking at one's function within the context of outcomes is a major psychological and behavioral shift in orientation. It should be expected to be a traumatic, challenging, and noisy transition.

The "tribal" orientation of both disciplines and departments creates natural barriers to the consideration of team-based relationships across the system. Increasingly, in building the continuum of care, integration between teams is as critical as integration within teams; therefore, in interdisciplinary team building, getting past the tribal consciousness will become critical to the success of the organization.

Every time we observe the organizational system, we can watch people and professions operating within the context of their own organizational structure and relationship, from providing service on units to eating lunch in the cafeteria. Understanding the phenomena associated with forming tribal groups and organizational bodies in interdisciplinary systems will be critical to dismantling them. Forming new relationships, liaisons, attachments, and organizational interactions will be critical to developing effective and sustainable team-based approaches.

Forming team-based relationships between and within teams along the continuum of care will be equally critical to the work of the organization. As more and more health care systems become integrated across patient pathways, building team-based relationships along those pathways will be as important as building team based relationships within the context of each team. Developing intersecting mechanisms, developing organizational and shared decision-making roles, and formatting organizational structures and governance frameworks for these more multifocal integrated systems will be important work of design.

When one attempts to build team-based organizational systems, the attempt leads to addressing all of the arenas of concern around the organizational system. No element of the organization, no component of structure, no design of the point-of-service or continuum can be addressed without looking at the other components of the organizational system and the impact each change has on the whole. When one begins to look at the interdisciplinary formation and nature of team-based design, it is clear that whole systems approaches must be incorporated into the view one brings to thinking about team-based approaches. Considerable focus and emphasis on critical design and structuring around the relationships disciplines have with each other will form the foundation for sustainable team-based formation and define the work in creating sustainable interdisciplinary teams.

FORCES INFLUENCING TEAM CONSTRUCTION

Many forces are at work in building interdisciplinary teams. Attention must be payed to integrating around value, the rules of relationship, and the unique and individualistic language of disciplines. There is a need for

TEAMTIP   4.3

Team Design Consistencies

1. The same principles of partnership, equity, accountability, and ownership govern all teams.
2. Teams are driven from their relationship with the patient, not their relationship with the system.
3. Teams focus on their work, which is guided by standards each member commits to.
4. Members are committed to building their relationships with each other, knowing that affects patient service.
5. Teams are places of continuous learning. Everyone is in development at all times and committed to continuous growth.
6. Teams are "we" places, not "I" places. The members seek to contribute their unique talents to the benefit of the team and to positively affect patients.

The single greatest challenge for the system attempting to build a team approach to work is the current compartmentalization of thinking and organizing. From CEO to provider, much of the work is changing thinking from vertical connections to horizontal relationships. Much of the success of the system will be based on its ability to make this change.

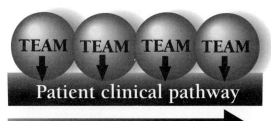

CLINICAL TEAM INTEGRATION

TEAM   TEAM   TEAM   TEAM

Patient clinical pathway

Patient's health journey

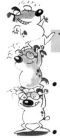

TEAMTIP   4.4

Basic Team Values

- *Each member is honored for his or her uniqueness and contribution.*
- *Every member contributes to the outcomes of the team.*
- *The team always addresses issues of conflict quickly and with good process.*
- *Dialogue is the central communication skill for team members.*
- *Teams are always evaluating the effectiveness of their work.*
- *Team activities are not fixed; they are changed as frequently as the demand for them changes.*
- *Teams' central purpose is meeting the needs of those they serve before any other consideration.*

common language, education, development, and shifting the professional mindset of each discipline; adjusting the thinking patterns that each discipline brings to the process; and altering the roles, relationships, and cultures that have developed within the context of each team. Bringing each of these unique sets of variables together under the umbrella of the integrated interdisciplinary team has imbedded in it a huge set of challenges (Team Tip 4-4). Much of the work of leadership will be in this arena. Most of the activities of creating effective interdisciplinary teams will be in the arena of sorting through the individual character of the disciplines and the application of individual disciplinary processes to an interdisciplinary framework.

Moving in the direction of creating interdisciplinary teams will require a huge educational effort. Indeed, much of what we identified as a part of a learning organization in Chapters 1 and 2 will be articulated in the process of developing interdisciplinary teams in a clinical environment. The stakeholders will need to be involved in design, in visioning, in construction of the transition and transformative process, in modeling and reinforcing new sets of behaviors, in development of new leadership and management processes in the organizational system, and in developing mechanisms for addressing the conflict that will invariably emerge in all of the efforts devoted to building an interdisciplinary mindset.

The movement away from notions of dependence and independence toward a level of interdependence will be a critical element of the process of building interdisciplinary teams (Team Tip 4-5). It is clear in all systems thinking that there really are no dependent or independent roles in human work groups; there are only interdependent roles that have imbedded in them individual as well as collective characteristics. The movement toward interdependence is the fundamental task and activity of work groups and leadership in building teams and team processes. Moving toward an interdependent organizational system (the team process) will require a clearly coordinated and well-defined developmental process. Developmental process should cover at least the following issues:

- A clear understanding of the meaning behind creating team-based approaches
- The basic concepts associated with team-based designs
- The terms of reference around building and constructing effective teams
- Point-of-service design and empowerment of staff members
- Full understanding of the change process and its impact on individual roles
- Interpersonal skill development and relationship building
- Identifying tribe behaviors and the shift toward interdependence
- The development of clearly enumerative communication and relational skills
- Collaboration/conflict resolution processes
- Building the process of dialogue in group dynamics

Each of these elements is a specific requisite of all disciplined team members on their way to understanding and incorporating team processes and behaviors into their own practices and processes. The organization's commitment to development, to understanding, to reskilling, and to changing the orientation of each member becomes a critical first step in ensuring that the interdisciplinary framework can be applied to team development in an effective and meaningful way.

The characteristics of interdependent and clinical teams in health care have many common characteristics with those of team development in

TEAMTIP   4-5

Moving toward Interdependence

In team-based approaches there are no independent or dependent functions. There are only interdependent actions. Each contribution by a team member is as important as that of another. Contribution is differentiated by role, not by importance of the person. This means:

- Equity between members is critical to good relationships.
- Working out personality problems is a high priority early in team relationships.
- Development of good problem-solving techniques in the team is important.
- Linking all clinical activities together ties team members to a common process and goal.
- Each member is valued for his or her contribution to the work of the team.

other service enterprises. However, health care is unique in the character and content of the discipline-specific approaches to delivering service. The disciplines have emerged as a part of the social mandate to protect the public and to provide a broad-based range of knowledge to a multiplicity of services in rendering health care to the community the professional serves. Honoring this unique contribution and the collective obligation all have to achieve higher levels of outcome becomes the critical cornerstone of team-based development.

The movement to bring professions together to create a common consciousness, a common commitment in an integrated approach to delivering point-of-service care is important in the next stage of health care maturation and refinement. Building service across the continuum of care,

The team will always be looking to create a real identity for itself to give members a sense of place and belonging in the larger system. All efforts of the team should be to make their relationship sustainable.

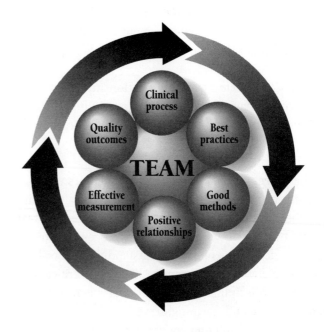

building subscriber-based pathways, and constructing service frameworks to support health rather than illness calls the disciplines together in a unique way. Developing the foundations for good team-based approaches will require much confrontation and noise in the system.

The challenge for each of the disciplines is the challenge for all of the disciplines. The commitment of all disciplines to the purpose of improving the health of individuals and society is at question in building team-based approaches. Crossing disciplinary parameters, moving from vertical orientation to horizontal linkages, creates a new demand on the disciplines to relate in a broader context and a deeper frame of reference. It challenges each discipline to test the value of its contribution against the outcomes of health each is required to obtain. It calls all the disciplines around the table to deal specifically with their common commitment, sort through their unique contribution, and, in the final analysis, identify that core, that common ground, to which each is committed in providing service and advancing the health of the community.

> *The work of all health professionals is to meet the needs of those they serve. Because they share the same commitment, they should be able to share the process.*

Bibliography

Bennis W, Biederman P: *Organizing genius,* New York, Addison-Wesley, 1997.

Graham M, Lebaron M: *The horizontal revolution: guiding the teaming takeover,* San Francisco, Jossey-Bass, 1994.

Janov J: *The inventive organization,* San Francisco, Jossey-Bass, 1994.

JHR Association: *Kaizen Teian 2,* Cambridge, Mass, Productivity Press, 1993.

Kottler J: *Beyond blame: a new way of resolving conflicts in relationship,* San Francisco, Jossey-Bass, 1996.

Lipman-Blumen J: *The connective edge: leading in an interdependent world,* San Francisco, Jossey-Bass, 1996.

Macy J: Collective self interest-the holonic shift, *World Business Academy Perspectives* 9(1):19-22, 1995.

Marcus L et al: *Renegotiating health care: resolving conflict to build collaboration,* San Francisco, Jossey-Bass, 1995.

Mason J: Building the team during consolidation, *Seminars for Nurse Managers* 2(4):213-217, 1994.

Meyer C: How the right measures help teams excel, *Harvard Business Review* 72(3):95-103, 1994.

Mohrman S, Cohen S, Mohrman A: *Designing team based organizations,* San Francisco, Jossey-Bass, 1995.

Mohrman S, Mohrman A: *Designing and leading team based organizations,* San Francisco, Jossey-Bass, 1997.

Neubauer J: Redesign: managing role changes and building a new team, *Seminars for Nurse Managers* 1(1):26-32, 1993.

Nirenberg J: *The living organization: transforming teams into workplace communities,* Homewood, Ill, Irwin Professional, 1993.

O'Hara Devereaux M, Johansen R: *Globalwork,* San Francisco, Jossey-Bass, 1994.

Pacanowsky M: Team tools for wicked problems, *Organizational Dynamics* 23(2):36-51, 1995.

Parker G: *Cross functional teams,* San Francisco, Jossey-Bass, 1994.

Parker G: *Team players and teamwork,* San Francisco, Jossey-Bass, 1996.

Pedersen A, Easton L: Teamwork: bringing order out of chaos, *Nursing Management* 26(6):34-35, 1995.

Perley MJ: Beyond shared governance: restructuring care delivery for self managed work teams, *Nursing Administration Quarterly* 19(1):12-20, 1994.

Schutz W: *The human element: workers and the bottom line,* San Francisco, Jossey-Bass, 1994.

Steckler N: Building team leader effectiveness: a diagnostic tool, *Organizational Dynamics* 23 (2):20-35, 1995.

Thompson C, Zondlo J: Building a case for team learning, *Health Care Forum Journal* 38(5):36-44, 1995.

Weisbord M: *Building common ground,* San Francisco, Barrett-Koehler, 1993.

Wilson J et al: *Leadership trapeze,* San Francisco, Jossey-Bass, 1994.

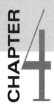

TOOLCHEST

TOOL A: Team Behavior Checklist

The following items are a pre-team checklist to help the facilitator focus on the individual team member's participation and involvement in the team process. This checklist helps the facilitator or team chairperson involve the team members fully in the issues of the team:

- All members are present.
- Each member knows the rules of engagement, which were shared at the beginning of the team session.
- Each member of the team has participated and shared his or her views during discussion.
- No team member was quiet.
- The facilitator asked direct questions to engage the more reflective participants.
- There are no hidden agendas.
- Each member is fully invested in the goals of the meeting.
- Every issue receives the attention it requires.
- There is no "acting out" by any member.
- Every discussion is reasonable and fact based.
- Personalities are not discussed nor attacked.

- People do not act out of anger.
- There is no side discussion or whispering occurring.
- Members are frank and open in their contributions to the discussion.
- Members feel generally good about the work and progress of the team meetings.
- The chairperson feels adequately supported by the members.
- The process of team meetings are orderly and progress well.
- Add additional needs:
  ....
  ....
  ....

The facilitator should attempt to review each of the sessions using this checklist and should add specific items to it that individualize evaluation to the demands of individual teams. This process will help keep the facilitator focused and aware of the impact of members on the team and identify problems that might arise during the team meetings.

TOOL B: Group Reality and Systems Exercise

This exercise has any permutations and sources but it is a good one to use at the beginning stages of group formation to lean quickly the dynamics of systems process within the context of a team process. It can be used for a group of up to 30 participants and is an excellent teacher of how groups can work well.

Tools: Three balls, preferably balls that do not bounce well.

Time: 30 minutes to one hour.

Instructions:

- Person must throw the ball to the same person each round and receive it from the same thrower each round, (the sender and receiver of the ball are different people).
- Whoever drops the ball must pick up his or her own ball.
- Throw the ball gently underhand.
- Place your hands in front of your body before you receive the ball and behind your body when you have completed your round.

Facilitator explains the above rules. Group is placed standing in a round circle facing in, with enough room between each participant to throw and receive a ball. The facilitator chooses a person who will always be the first tosser. The exercise is explained, and the participants are told they will be timed regarding how long it will take to complete throwing and receiving the ball by each member around the circle. The goal is to toss the ball completely to each member in as efficient and timely a fashion as possible. The facilitator is trying to obtain the best time and usually allows three cycles of throwing to get the best time with the ball.

After completing the best time run with one ball around the circle the facilitator introduces a second ball into the exercise to be thrown around the participant circle in the same order and manner as the first ball. This too is timed and compared to the time of throwing one ball. The same is done with a third ball. Each ball is generally given three rounds to get the best time. Outcomes obtained in this exercise include the following:

- The times for throwing three balls are close to the same as the time for throwing one ball.
- The participant get better at throwing and timing the balls.
- A pattern of flow between participants and balls begins to emerge.
- The teamwork begins to become strong and effective.
- Other individual patterns of systems affecting the team becomes clear to team members.

An evaluation of the process with individual debriefing should occur right after the exercise, with a focus on the implications this exercise has for creating team relationships, effectiveness, and outcomes. Some rules of team behavior and functioning should flow from the debriefing session. This is a good exercise to do periodically to help re-engage team members to what is necessary to ensure good team process and successful team relationships.

5

The Manager's Role in a Team-Based System

If people were always to speak their mind on issues both great and small, they would be considered insubordinate by the average supervisor and a threat to an organization.

M. Scott Peck

Managers are no longer called on to direct people but to manage the systems that support people managing themselves. The unprecedented movement to point-of-service, multidisciplinary, and clinically-based team systems creates a significant demand for changes in the manager's function and role. The manager's role in a team-based system is that of a facilitator who stimulates teams to action in capable ways. This behavioral change creates a tremendous impact on the requisite abilities of managers to move from hierarchical models into team-based systems. The characteristics of a team-based system are summarized in Box 5-1.

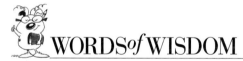

WORDS *of* WISDOM

The biggest problem in health care organization today is not health care reform, but the human ego. We will fail in our efforts if we do not get out of our own way.

$\sim$

BOX **5-1**

Traditional vs. Team-Based Organizations	
TRADITIONAL	TEAM BASED
Management driven	Patient centered
Isolated specialists	Multifunction workers
Job descriptions	Performance competencies
Many layers	Flattened management
Department focus	Continuum focus
Management control	Team direction
Policy procedure driven	Value and process driven
Top-down appraisals	360-degree appraisals
Tightly organized	Sometimes chaotic

Adapted from Bergman TJ, DeMeuse KP: Diagnosing whether an organization is truly ready to empower work team: a case study, *Human Resource Planning* 19(1):38-48, 1996.

FOCUS

Some Symptoms of Sick Organizations
- Decisions are based on rumor and whispers.
- Employees feel oppressed and vulnerable.
- Rewards are tied to "who you know."
- People are masters at avoiding risk.
- There is a strong undertone of anger and fear.

MOVING TO A TEAM-BASED ORGANIZATION

A major problem facing American caregivers is not "burnout" from overwork but a crisis of constant and gross underutilization of worker potential (Ghashal and Bartle, 1996). Caregivers in realigned organizations cannot be made to feel valuable and empowered, they simply *are*. The behavioral context of work is experienced in the "feel" of the place. Does your organization feel fresh and crisp, with a certain eagerness to experiment? Or is it oppressive and polluted with anger, anxieties, and fear of the unknown? The former is invigorating; the latter will wear people down. The pathologies of our inherited conduct make this work challenging. Health care organizations come from a tradition of excessive control and compliance, which must be replaced in a team-based system with contracts, partnership, accountability, support, and stretching the limits.

WE REALLY HAVE NO NEED FOR MANAGERS ANYWAY; OR DO WE?

Organizations need management practices more than ever, but not in the old way. The manager in a team-based system is a designer, teacher, facilitator, and steward.

People can tolerate the uncertainty of today's environment, accepting both hard work and hard choices, when they have the systems and processes that support working and meeting challenges together.

The business rationale for teams is simple. Changes in the health care marketplace have led organizations to look at the implementation of team-based systems as work design and human resource strategies. Management teams that pursue this approach maximize organizational flexibility, attract and sustain highly skilled and responsive staff, and enhance the use of information in data-driven decision making (Jenkins, 1994).

For people to move beyond the threats of downsizing, reorganized workplaces, or new relationships, management must create work environments where there is an emphasis on continuous self-renewal in the service of others. This requires significant trust. In a rapidly changing and competitive marketplace, trust in the workplace is essential because it translates directly into productivity.

The manager's role in team-based systems is different and much more challenging: to drive fear out of the workplace; hold sacred the values, beliefs, and goals of service; design processes that create a humane workplace; and look for opportunities to facilitate learning in the pursuit of outcomes.

PEOPLE ARE ENVIRONMENT

However, to maximize individual and team performance, strategies cannot be limited to simply revamping processes or changing organizational structures. *The most vital focal points for transformation are the actions and behaviors of individual people and groups.* Failing to understand this basic premise

The degree to which the context of work is exhilarating in health care organizations is a direct outcome of the invisible hands of managers.

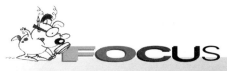

What Managers Need to Handle for Teams

- *Workflow and timing problems*
- *Conflict vs. team leader and manager role*
- *Unclear authority*
- *Limiting amount of formalization (rigidity)*
- *Opportunities for reflection*

has led to the demise of many a change project. Managing behavior is central to the development of team-based systems. The behaviors of organization members not only shape the organization's internal culture but also the quality of the organization's external relationships.

The wise manager will consider several implications to this strategy before plunging ahead and developing teams.

Implication #1: The Gap

There is always a gap between how staff members and top management perceive the concept of moving to teams (Holpp, 1996). Staff members usually welcome the freedom that comes with teams: to implement controls over their own work and to have the authority to solve problems at the point-of-service. On the other hand, top management see the implementation of teams as a competitive strategy. Teams are expected to put the goal of the organization above the needs of the individual. Personal sacrifices will be made on behalf of the team. Also, the expectation that teams will create greater productivity may lead top executives to assume that there will be a downsizing of staff in the future. When these outcomes are not immediately apparent, executives may become disillusioned with teams and withdraw their support.

Closing the gap

This gap is the widest in early implementation. After the initial "honeymoon" period, staff members' behaviors may signal dissatisfaction with the team and anxiety about the possibility of layoffs. Executives may question the wisdom of moving forward. The amount of conflict generated by these two different perspectives can be minimized if, early on, teams make a valued contribution to the organization's goals and are assisted by managers who remove the obstacles that interfere with doing a good job.

If teams are not well supported, they will remain ineffective grafts to a hierarchical structure, fail to achieve outcomes, and be perceived as a drain on the organization's resources. Slowly but surely, parallel processes will be created to get work done despite the teams. These duplicative methods operate outside the team structure and eventually overcome the team.

Staff members need to know what the human resources policy is should productivity improve and layoffs follow. Will people be afforded the opportunity to apply for other positions in the system? Will they be given the training to pursue different jobs? Following is an example of how managers react in a potential layoff situation.

One hospital provided a college-credited public health nursing course to associate degree nurses who wanted to avoid potential layoff by moving into the new home health nursing program (San Antonio et al., 1995). This approach signaled to the workforce that management valued their contributions to the organization and was seeking ways to maximize employment opportunities for the workforce in the face of declining revenues. Fixing the bottom line was not the only focus of this management team.

Managers typically believe that staff members will work more and harder because of commitment to team goals. Staff members typically believe that teams will result in work being easier. Shared definitions of the team's work must precede implementation.

If these issues are not anticipated and addressed, the gap between managers' and staff members' expectations will remain wide, and the behavior will be disruptive. People might agree on the *value* of a team-based organization but disagree about what a team-based organization *is*.

Implication #2: Imprisonment

Organizations must have the potential to learn, unlearn, or relearn based on their experiences. Many managers remain prisoners of outdated mental maps (Niccolini et al., 1995). Can every member of the management team draw the same process map for the organization? For organizations to be aligned with their internal and external environments, managers must learn, unlearn, and relearn their mental models of work in health care organizations.

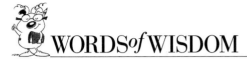

WORDS of WISDOM

Beware of those who say that they support teams but fail to provide the necessary meeting time, schedule adjustments, or management of sudden increases in census or overtime.
These people do not support their teams!

~

Management defines the potential impact of layoffs on teams and the labor force before implementing such action.

There is agreement about how much work is expected of team members.

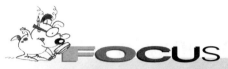

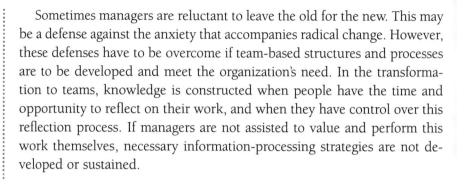

WORDS of WISDOM

A most important consideration in the implementation process is your patience!

⁓

Sometimes managers are reluctant to leave the old for the new. This may be a defense against the anxiety that accompanies radical change. However, these defenses have to be overcome if team-based structures and processes are to be developed and meet the organization's need. In the transformation to teams, knowledge is constructed when people have the time and opportunity to reflect on their work, and when they have control over this reflection process. If managers are not assisted to value and perform this work themselves, necessary information-processing strategies are not developed or sustained.

Avoiding imprisonment

The social construction of new knowledge in organizations is a powerful management tool in the implementation of teams. It leads to shared knowledge, shared meanings, and a predominant definition of the way to be and do in the new order of things. If learning does not occur, the necessary new knowledge to do the new work is not created.

Implication #3: Power

The empowerment of teams cannot be directed by the executive level without a corresponding movement of power (O'Leary, 1996). Teams are effective in those workplaces where work requires a combination of expertise and when cross-functional problem solving is required.

The delivery of quality health care services demands the cooperation of many people. To successfully develop teams, you must recognize that the change process is more than saying "Let's just do it!" Some people erroneously believe the change process resembles the purchase of a piece of capital equipment or turning on a light. Strong project management takes care of the tasks. An understanding and a facilitation of the human side of change management takes care of the process side.

As the traditional doers and fixers in the organization, managers must now demonstrate the forbearance to wait 3 to 5 years for sustainable outcomes. In the meantime, all members of management must examine infrastructure, policies, and procedures that focus on the individual, and modify them to support the team structure or eliminate the potential for individual power trips. There is more than enough management work to be done as teams take the time to fully develop their effectiveness.

Moving power

Before implementing teams, managers must be clear about the fact that some of their authority will indeed be transferred to teams. The examination of authority boundaries is a critical step. The team chartering process described in Chapter 8 assists with this process. For some managers, authority and accountability for the point-of-service care will be difficult to transfer to teams. This is because in team-based systems, managers are held accountable for exercising their authority in relationship to business operations. Some managers do not have such skill.

Implication #4: Communication

The quality of interactions in teams is higher than that in traditional work groups. The quality and level of team interactions are directly related to team effectiveness (Cashman, 1995). To successfully meet their objectives, teams must develop new and effective patterns of communication that did not occur when the manager made the decisions. This is a paradox for managers.

Managers are compelled to unlearn past ways of communicating and to encourage their replacement with team communication systems. Obstacles that have been built over time are often difficult to see. Therefore managers will participate in rather than lead team-building activities, so as to strengthen team communication systems. Team building, discussed in greater detail in Chapter 3, is a prerequisite in the development of the peer-directed communication of teams if group decision making and consensus are to replace the decision-making role of the manager.

Effective lateral relationships are a hallmark of team-based organizations. These interaction patterns contribute to or detract from the effec-

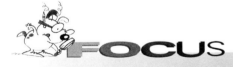

Peer-Directed Communication

Feedback
Interpretation of events
Assistance
Respect for ideas
Quality exchanges
Role expectations
Modification and testing of present roles

tiveness of teams. Some teams, through their negative intrateam relationships, have efficiently fish-boned a problem while lessening the quality of the final decision,

Have you experienced times when you acted in a considerate fashion toward the team, but team members remained dissatisfied? Why? The explanation centers on the *quality of the interaction* between leaders and followers. Even the most effective manager can be confronted with dysfunctional teams who engage in stalling, quiet sabotage, communication failure, or poor decision making because of team relationships. Traditional management communication focuses on the economic self interest of followers, while managers who focus on interactions seek to elevate partners to new levels of commitment, integrity, and quality. Although there are managers who can and do operate in the context of interaction and relationships, many corporate health care structures have continued to train and reward only the traditional command and control models of management.

Relationship-based management

Relationship-based management behaviors are central to successful management in a team-based organization. Management behaviors have a powerful impact on the culture of the organization. Teams reconstruct their beliefs, habits, or work rituals because they internalize the values of the organization. The manager is the organization's representative. Relationship-based managers transform themselves, teams of caregivers, and therefore their organizations through mutually empowering relationships (Sashkin, 1984).

Hence, relationship-centered management is an ethical process between leaders and followers. Instead of self-involvement, control, and power wielding, leaders' actions are not separate and distinct from followers' needs and goals. Such managers work with groups to develop mutually agreed-on goals, look at the actual work being performed, and put those who are performing the work into decision-making roles regarding their work. These strategies stress the importance of shared goals over the leader's desires.

Identifying the "types" of team behaviors is not the same as understanding the patterns of interaction within and between teams.

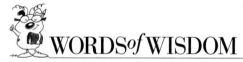

WORDS*of*WISDOM

A collision with the interdependent management style of team-based systems is inevitable, so be prepared to manage the politics!

～

Implication #5: Cost

Teamwork is not easy, nor is it without cost (O'Leary, 1996). Groups of individuals do not become teams because they are directed to do so. Building effective teams requires the provision of considerable resources such as formal management development for new roles, conflict resolution skills, management of group dynamics, and consensus decision-making tools (Box 5-2). Team skill development is a learning process that takes time and experience. Early ventures into team decision making may produce struggles and team frustration, and people can become disenchanted with teamwork.

Managers will need to "keep the faith" by reinforcing the value of teamwork to avoid low morale and loss of productivity. To act as cheerleaders, managers must believe that, in the long run, teams will produce better decisions and greater productivity. The following is an example of the effects of management decision making.

Executive management implemented self-managed teams as a productivity measure. Emphasis on the bottom line resulted in few resources being provided to assist people to work in teams. Decision making was laborious. Executives responded with "crisis" decisions outside of the team structure. Soon, the majority of organizational decisions were being made in this crisis mode. A consultant was then hired to develop the managers in team leadership practices. Halfway through the first leadership training session, the agenda had to be dropped because of angry participants. A large group intervention revealed that the participants were angry with top management for implementing the team concept and then not supporting it. They felt blamed for their teams' failures and constrained in their developmental work by fiscal limitations. The last thing that the participants wanted to hear was that they were to be cheerleaders. A management retreat produced consensus about definitions, accountabilities, outcomes, and the resources needed to support self-managed teams in the context of this organization's resources.

The essence of the manager-staff relationship is the interaction between differences in the goals, motivation, skill set, and influence potential of every stakeholder.

BOX **5-2**

Resources Needed by Teams

- Team training
- Dedicated meeting time
- Personal space and office supplies (team room)
- A defined budget
- An active facilitator
- Library access to support data-driven decisions
- Management support

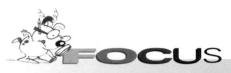

Questions of Cost and Feasibility

- Are work processes compatible with teams?
- Are employees willing and able to make teams work?
- Can managers master and apply shared leadership?
- Is your market healthy enough to support increased productivity without layoffs?
- Do we really want teams?

Anticipating cost

To help anticipate cost, managers should establish a budget for the project, establish budgets for teams and hold them accountable for outcomes, and approach the evaluation of cost-effectiveness from the value-added perspective.

Demonstrating the cost-effectiveness of team-based systems through traditional methods is difficult. Managers commonly err by trying to count the number of committees replaced or the time spent in meetings before and after implementation of a team-based system, but these are not useful measures because they do not measure contribution. Instead, it is useful to examine the value-added contributions made by teams when

1. Structures, systems, and processes are standardized.
2. Errors are reduced.
3. Productivity is enhanced.
4. High-volume, high-cost, problem-prone quality issues are improved.

Implication #6: Ripple Effects

Team decision making and team projects cause ripple effects across the organization. Shared decision making requires a major paradigm shift for managers and staff. The cultural and political impacts of moving to a team-based system should not be diminished.

There will always be people—executives, middle managers, and staff members—who do not welcome changes in control, autonomy, or accountability. If the implementation of teams is not managed well, these issues can build significant cultural resistance and will threaten the delicate imbedding of teams in the organization.

Reducing ripple effects

The ripple effect can be reduced by knowing who is "on board" and who is not. Anticipate the reactions of influential stakeholders in instances where the noise of change is high or when mistakes have been made. Act decisively to intervene. If possible, convert the circumstances to a win-win

WORDS of WISDOM

This ripple feels more like a riptide!

120

situation by including the useful perspectives of unsupportive stakeholders in problem resolution. Keep the issue of nonsupportive stakeholders on the public agenda, so that organizational interventions can be considered and implemented to reduce their resistance.

MANAGEMENT SERVICES FOR TEAMS

Five groundwork activities are critical in supporting the development of effective teams (Ehlen, 1994): (1) develop vision alignment; (2) build shared accountability; (3) provide individual, as well as team, development; (4) support mutual influence; and (5) build task autonomy.

Develop Vision Alignment

Efforts to implement teams must be clearly tied to the organization's strategies. Without this connection, staff can make up their own reasons. Whatever the reason for implementing teams, it should be stated clearly and in practical terms. Vision is a tool used to inspire people to go the extra mile, to correct misperceptions, and the obstacles they present. A clear vision also assists management and clinical leaders to articulate what is exciting or challenging about working in the organization.

Build Shared Accountability

The team itself has accountability for its own experience. Teams are made up of diverse people with unique skills, interests, and beliefs. However, some groups mistakenly believe that individual differences must be forsaken in the face of the team's decision. This erroneous belief leads to dysfunctional team behaviors such as "groupthink," in which people withhold their true opinions because of perceived peer pressure (Harvey, 1988). High-performing teams use the unique contributions of individuals to achieve shared goals. This spirit of collaboration permits members to constructively confront the differences among them.

One method of retaining individual differences while working on a team is the team accountability contract found at the end of this chapter. This

121

BOX 5-3

Objectives of a "Train-the-Trainer" Program

At the end of the train-the-trainer workshop(s), participants will be able to do the following:

1. Describe the components of a systems approach to leadership development.
2. Apply concepts of behavioral learning to selected workshops for leadership training.
3. Define a shared leadership development program that can be implemented in the participants' home organization.

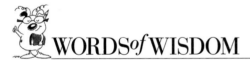

WORDS*of*WISDOM

If I can do it, you can too!

tool assists members in expressing their feelings and making decisions as a team. This exercise has additional benefit in that it clearly places accountability for the team's dynamics in the hands of team members. Team members discuss what a particular accountability statement means to them. They then have the actual experience of retaining their identity to move the group to completion of its work. This experience reinforces belief in the team's capability to make key decisions jointly.

Provide Individual, as Well as Team, Development

Team potential can be developed at every level so that each individual has the maximum capability to contribute. This can be achieved through informal coaching and facilitation and strengthened by formal team development programs. The development of peer communications can also be strengthened when a "train the trainer" approach is used to carry learning to all parts of the system. Once organizations have completed shared leadership training, there is often a need to provide additional workshops as new people are hired or for additional groups of staff. In this workshop, the trainer assists the organization in developing modules of shared leadership workshops, using a train-the-trainer methodology (see Box 5-3).

Multidisciplinary groups of staff members, educators, and managers work with the trainer to develop a systematic approach to a leadership program, which is owned and implemented by the organization. Internal trainers are taught principles of behavioral learning, a systems approach to leadership development, and the rationale underlying selected workshops. In this instance, a core group of trainers is developed in just-in-time and behavioral learning methodologies. After they have completed a core program of shared leadership skill development, they are assisted in the development of modules, which they then teach to various teams. As internal trainers provide this training for new team roles, they become expert themselves in the shared leadership skills, which is an added benefit to team development. In addition, there is considerable cost savings to the organization. Expensive training programs can be limited to a core group, followed by a fluid and dynamic team of internal trainers who take the training across the system.

Support Mutual Influence

One of the first steps in building influence is to encourage team members to disagree with a person holding a leadership role in the organization. This experience can be a cathartic experience for individuals, as they experience the validation of shared decision making as a part of their actual work experience. We have heard individuals repeatedly tell stories of a particular moment in time when they became "true believers." Never underestimate the power of a positive (or negative) cathartic moment. Consider these comments made by an operating room nurse in an organization implementing a team-based system:

"I have been at this hospital for over 20 years, and I have seen a lot of things come and go. When I first heard about this project, I was pretty skeptical. Words are fine but you don't know what it's really like to work here. Anyway, when we were able to confront the V.P. of Patient Care Services about how poorly the downsizing was going and how it was affecting our teams ... I was amazed! Not only did he sit and listen but he actually asked our advice. He asked the staff's opinion! He even implemented some of our suggestions. From then on, I knew we were really going to change. That is when I got committed. Now no one can convince me any differently."

Build Task Autonomy

Encourage teams to consult their own experts. You might provide names, but it is up to the team to engage such people, insist on their support, and request specific information. In the beginning, teams may be wary of approaching people who hold positions of influence in the organization, such as the hospital attorney or the director of case management. Remember that the quality of the team's decisions are only as good as their information.

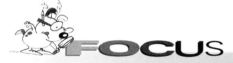

Creating a Team Player Culture

- *Promote only team players*
- *Top executives model team player role*
- *360-degree appraisals*
- *Define team player competencies*
- *Hiring evaluates for team competencies*

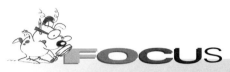

When Should Managers Intervene?

Managers should intervene quickly when:

- *Negative politics are at play (e.g., manipulation).*
- *The team is adrift.*
- *The grapevine communicates negative individual behaviors.*
- *The team is stuck in bureaucratic gridlock.*

BOX 5-4

Example from the Field

The vice president of a large hospital surrounded herself with people like herself who were experts at PERT charts and the linear thinking that accompanies their application. Unfortunately, it took forever for anything to get done because of the time spent in analysis, and there was little tolerance for divergent thinking. Teams kept such thoughts to themselves. The "how to be" manager continually performs a "mirror test," asking "Am I the person that I want to be? Am I modeling successful behaviors?"

Intervene only when all efforts to engage the expert have proven unsuccessful. You know that you are dealing with a different problem altogether when this happens.

BECOMING A "HOW TO BE" LEADER

Past knowledge of people and systems is of little help to the manager interested in creating a new behavioral context for work. Instead, the source of wisdom comes from one's own self-observations and the purposeful modeling of expected new behaviors. It is not news that managers are expected to be role models; however, the focal point has changed. The emphasis is no longer on teaching people how to *do* but how to *be*. The "how to be" manager inspires followers, is respected for results, is highly visible, and sets clear behavioral examples of leadership. These leaders see their role not as rank or privilege but as a responsibility to the caregiver. They ask "What needs to be done?" rather than "What do I want?" This question is accompanied by clear definitions of what constitutes both results and poor performance.

The like or dislike of people or personalities is no longer an issue, because such leaders recognize that complex health care organizations demand diversity in leadership if performance is to be strong (Box 5-4).

Health care organizations hold a preoccupation with leadership, as well as with the ambivalence with which it is viewed. The yearning for decisive leaders and the apprehension that they might upset the balance between power and autonomy have made us more adept at demanding leadership than truly embracing it.

THE SPECIAL CASE OF EXECUTIVE TEAMS

Top management teams perceive, interpret, and act on their environments in a manner different from the management team as a whole. The interpretive dynamics of executive teams must be understood and evaluated in times of drastic change. The dynamics of top teams are instrumental in how they experience the environment and how those perceptions are translated into strategic and operational actions. The degree of confidence executive teams have in their organization's strategic direction is a significant trust factor that emerges in times of change. Managers' behaviors, including patience, tolerance for the slowness or speed of change, response to errors, and willingness to trust, are all influenced by this certainty about organizational direction. To make matters worse, members of the team may not have the same level of comfort or discomfort. Four factors can influence the level of certainty executive teams have with the organizational direction of a team-based system:

1. *Amount of environmental volatility.* Turbulence creates anxiety stemming from uncertainty about the future in general or one's own career in particular. Excessive anxiety diminishes tolerance for any additional instability.

2. *Comfort with consensus.* If the executive team is not cohesive in the first place, they cannot pull together to face their collective environmental challenges and almost certainly will have trouble being united in support of change. When executive teams are together, they produce better coordinated actions, which in turn contribute to their own sense of certainty and self-effectiveness.

3. *Degree of satisfaction with the executive team.* Is there a strong team orientation, or do members operate as independent contractors of functional departments? Do interactions reflect patterns of trust, respect for each other's contributions, and collaboration in the pursuit of organizational goals? If the answer is no, the change to team-based systems will be fraught with difficulties in team dynamics because of inadequate role models. Also, lack of respect for the team by executive team members contributes to uncertainty because of inability to trust the team's decisions.

4. *Degree of knowledge about the health care environment.* Formal information and mental models shape executive action. How accurate is your executive team's perception of the health care environment? The accuracy of these perceptions affects the degree of confidence executives

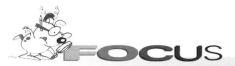

A Checklist for the "How to Be" Manager

- *Do your words and behavior consistently express belief that people are the greatest asset?*
- *Do you build diverse leaders and disperse the leadership of clones?*
- *Are you intolerant of poor performance?*
- *Do you know how to mobilize people with a clear sense of direction and the opportunity to find meaning in work?*
- *Can you listen to people and learn what they value?*
- *Do your values include a healthy sense of community?*
- *Are you able to rejoice in the strengths of associates?*
- *Can you tolerate not being popular but being right?*

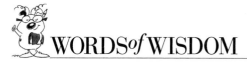

WORDS of WISDOM

It is no joke—leaders must be able to be taken seriously.

~

have in feeling that they understand what is going on and are confident that they can act effectively to respond to challenges. If perceptions are inaccurate, executive teams will struggle with the business case for moving to team-based systems.

Executive teams are well advised to take the time to retreat together and explore some of the following questions *before* the implementation of a team-based system:

- What is the biggest mistake that we made in the last 12 months? How did this happen?
- What does that mistake demonstrate about our team character, dynamics, and performance?
- What were the main criticisms leveled at you by your boss, your colleagues, your staff members, or your customers the last time your work as a team was examined?
- What is your greatest strength as a manager? What is your biggest problem?
- Can you think of any reason why this executive team might improve?
- When was the last time this executive team sat down and analyzed its own job performance?
- Is your team realistic? Can you face up to your problems? Can you admit to shortcomings? Do you recognize when you, not the staff, are the problem? Can you admit mistakes?
- When things go wrong, do you blame each other, circumstances, or bad luck?
- Do you like being members of this particular team of people?
- Does membership in this executive team contribute to your success in this organization?
- What do you intend to do with the information that you have learned from each other today?

Bibliography

Bergman TJ, DeMeuse, KP: Diagnosing whether an organization is truly ready to empower work teams: a case study, *Human Resource Planning* 19(1):38-48, 1996.

Cashman JF: Team member exchange under team and traditional management groups: a naturally occurring quasi-experiment study, *Group and Organizational Management* 20(1):18-39, 1995.

Ehlen D: Supporting high performance teams, *Manage* 46(2):32-35, 1994.

Ghoshal S, Bartlett C: Rebuilding behavioral context: a blueprint for corporate renewal, *Sloan Management Review* 37(2):23-37, 1996.

Harvey JB: *The Abilene paradox and other meditations on management,* San Diego, Pfeiffer & Co, 1988, pp 13-37.

Holpp L: The betrayal of the American work team: a fable of sorts, *Training* 33(5):38-42, 1996.

Isabella A, Waddock SA: Top management team certainty: environmental assessments, teamwork and performance implications, *Journal of Management* 20(4):835-859, 1994.

Jenkins A: Teams: from ideology to analysis, *Organizational Studies* 15(6):849-861, 1994.

Kennedy MM: The politics of intervention, *Across the Board* 31(9):11-13, 1994.

O'Leary L: Do you really need a team? *National Productivity Review* 15(4):1-5, 1996.

Niccolini D et al: The social construction of organizational learning: conceptual and practical issues of the field, *Human Relations* 48(7):729-747, 1995.

San Antonio AM et al: Consortium program prepares nurses for shift to community-based nursing, *Aspens Advisor for Nurse Executives* 10(12):7-8, 1995.

Sashkin M: Participative management is an ethical imperative, *Organizational Dynamics* (3):4-22, Spring 1984.

Tresolini CP, The Pew-Fetzer Task Force: *Health professions education and relationship-centered care,* San Francisco, Fetzer Institute and Pew Health Profession Commission, 1994.

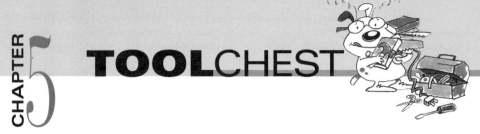

TOOLCHEST

TOOL A: Setting Group Guidelines: An Accountability Contract

Instructions: With your work group, review these guidelines. Delete any that are not appropriate. Adapt any to fit your needs, or write new ones. When the group reaches consensus, each member signs the agreement.

1. We will be as open as possible but honor the right of privacy.
2. What is discussed in our group will remain confidential.
3. We will respect differences. We will not discount others' ideas.
4. We will be supportive rather than judgmental.
5. We will give feedback directly and openly, and it will be given in a timely fashion. We will provide information that is specific and focused on the task and process and not personalities.
6. Within our group, we have the resources needed to solve any problem that arises. This means that we will all be contributors, sharing our unique perspective.

7. We are each responsible for what we get from this group experience. We will ask for what we need from our facilitator and the other group members.
8. We will try to get better acquainted with each other so we can identify ways in which we can develop professionally.
9. We will use our time well, be on time for work, and end our meetings promptly.
10. When members miss a meeting, we will share the responsibility to fill them in.
11. We will keep our focus on our goals, avoiding personality conflicts, hidden agendas, and getting sidetracked. We will acknowledge problems and deal with them.
12. We will not make phone calls or interrupt the group.

Group signatures:

Effective Teams Begin with the Self

Life in the organization may feel like a game of pinball but it works more like the human body . . . maybe we are an important part like manager of the heart.

Barry Oshry

Managers, unfortunately, can fall into the habit of repeating themselves over and over, for fear of venturing out into new territory. When the new territory finally comes, it may be too late to change, resulting in being at risk for out-placement. Although change is frightening, there is no alternative. Power in organization is being redefined. Employees are gaining access to information that once was monopolized by management. As wisdom is being redistributed to all levels of the organization, so is influence. The employee needs to be out there, more visible, more committed to teaching others what change is all about. It is not as easy as it seems.

The notion of "teamwork" creates a paradox for many managers. It is exceedingly difficult to subordinate some of the past freedoms imbedded in the traditional supervisory role. A manager must let go of the freedom to act on personal drive and achievement, placing himself secondary to the desires of a team. If this fails, however, the manager may find himself being labeled as an "obstructionist." In the final analysis, those who struggle with team-based management practices often move inconsistently from no leadership to micromanagement.

What is the alternative? Those managers who are successful in the transition to team-based organization are able to lift their thinking from indi-

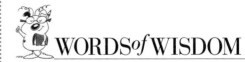

WORDS *of* WISDOM

Fear is not your enemy but your friend. It keeps you alive and alert in these challenging times. Fear offers you the chance to keep growing and to create in the midst of chaos. To manage you must take risks.

~

vidual to team outcomes. They confront the ghosts of their past, including old baggage with other people. They understand the difference between negative and positive politics; the former hurts people while the latter recognizes differences in influence. These leaders have also learned how not to be burned up by anxiety. Hence, they do not waste energy in hand-wringing and complaints. They know that their success is deeply imbedded in the success of other people. Because of these characteristics, successful managers in team-based organizations are more optimistic about the future and are committed to activities beyond their own ego needs. As one manager so fittingly described her journey:

"I am now seeing my life as one, long, ongoing process of self-discovery, rather than a series of promotions. The journey is clearly unpredictable. I know now that I cannot really control what will happen. Our organization, its processes, and its people are just too complex for that! So, I have to continually engage in a dialogue with myself about my own potential, what am I here for, and the realities of my current work situation."

A CRISIS OF SELF-ESTEEM IN LEADERSHIP

Contemplation and the willingness to state one's reflections in the public arena require leaders with a particular kind of courage and a strong sense of self. One of the marvels of the human personality is its resistance to prediction. We have observed in our work that one executive's paralyzing trauma is another person's invitation to take control of his or her life. One person's grounds for insanity can be another person's dramatic reshaping of the self (Blanchard, 1996).

To sustain healthy work environments in times of drastic change, health care managers must be able to see and act on the relationship of self-esteem and work, *beginning with themselves!*

The American work week, which shrunk to 40 hours in 1973, is back up to 46 hours per week. There are 10 fewer hours of leisure time per week, as compared with 15 years ago (Schor, 1992). Work dominates healthcare managers' lives and can consume over two thirds of their day.

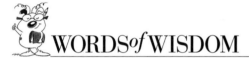

WORDS *of* WISDOM

One person's grounds for insanity can be another person's dramatic reshaping of the self. It's up to you!

~

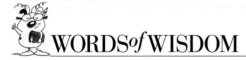

WORDS *of* WISDOM

You can choose to see your life positively or negatively—and if you choose the latter, chances are your self-esteem is not too great.

~

Not only are we working harder, but our work environments are making many of us sick. Health care, unfortunately, is no exception. What is the quality of your work relationships? Workplaces are traumatized by executives who manipulate to win, no matter what the human cost. They fail to act on the hard work of their people and operate from a perspective where only their objectives count. Accompanying this demoralizing style are often countless short-term fixes, which ultimately erode the very mission of the organization. Such management practices are the source of sleepless nights, migraine headaches, ulcers, and even heart attacks for many of their employees. These managers do not seem to be aware of the impact that they are having on others, when it should be readily apparent that the organization is suffering.

MANAGER BEHAVIORS THAT THREATEN TEAM PRODUCTIVITY*

Verbal Assaults to Self-Esteem

Managers with a negative view of people are both distrustful of others and suspicious of their motives. For example, questions posed to team members can be designed to uncover mistakes: "Do you mean to say that you didn't circulate that memo until yesterday? How will people be prepared?" Or "Oh, I see; you did not know that that quality improvement project would have an impact on your objectives." Under the guise of helpfulness, these types of critical interactions serve only to dishearten team members.

Talking Down to People

In this case, insecure managers communicate in such a way as to reinforce their superior position in the hierarchy. Some may even continue to emphasize this superiority, despite the fact that the hierarchy has been dis-

*Cyr R: Maintaining employee self-esteem, *Supervisory Management* 37(6):1-3, 1992.

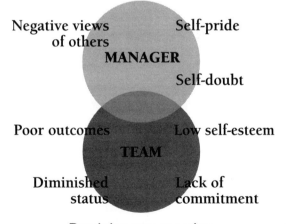

SELF-ESTEEM TRAP IN TEAM-BASED ORGANIZATION

Low self-esteem

Negative views of others

Self-pride

MANAGER

Self-doubt

Poor outcomes

Low self-esteem

TEAM

Diminished status

Lack of commitment

Passivity or nonaction

mantled! "*My* staff knows *my* way of doing business. *I* know ways to get things done around here that *they* could not possibly learn." Patronizing interaction destroys dignity and reinforces the "we-they" relationships of managers to staff.

Dictating Choices

Here, vulnerable managers can foster team dependency and delay action by providing the team with alternative choices for action. Providing the answers is not coaching but directing. A directive style simply fosters the learned passivity of most people in organizations. Early in a team's development, managers may need to more directly assist the team with exploring suggested alternatives. If the manager remains in this role, the team will never assume accountability for its own actions. When the manager is the team's parent, team members enact childlike behaviors. Because children fear punishment for their mistakes, they will avoid this discomfort by delegating all accountability upward . . . to the manager (Maccoby, 1993).

Petty Criticisms of Major Accomplishments

This constellation of behaviors in the insecure manager is expressed in a series of fault-finding and micromanagement activities. A most frequent place for such managers to aim and successfully fire is in the organizational process of communicating changes. Any person who has led a major change process is aware that no matter how many different ways information is communicated, there are employees who "never heard this before." This is a golden moment for the micromanager, who insists that teams eat up their valuable time recommunicating information that some people will never accept. When such criticism follows hollow praise for past communication efforts, it diminishes the team's efforts, prevents the team from moving on its objectives, and can make team members question their own potential for contribution.

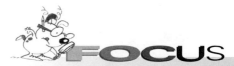

FOCUS

Four Management Reasons for not Giving too Much Information

- It will only upset and worry staff members.
- If I level with people they might level with me.
- It is their job to find out what they need.
- People need to concentrate on their own job and not on what someone else is doing.

Leaving Things Unsaid

An uncertain manager habitually hoards information as a power tool. Uncomfortable in the team setting, their actions surrounding information can be problematic. They may start to share information and then cut themselves off for "sharing too much." They may leave the room during important discussions to take phone calls or answer pages. Their nonverbal behavior may convey that they know something about the topic but are unwilling to share it. Such actions insult the team and strongly communicate that the manager is not open to the exchange of information or feedback on the information.

Denigrating the Importance of an Activity

All of us identify to some degree with our job. Team members enact this dynamic when they connect to the goals of the team. Significant energy is expended to attain quality outcomes. Managers with low self-esteem can lower the importance of this work, as well as the team's perception of its status in the organization. "Well, some people feel you are spending too much time doing this work, instead of patient care."

Carrying a Grudge

Clearly, a member of an organization for any length of time will have a history with another member, characterized by dissatisfaction or disappointment. Employees are extremely sensitive to manager disapproval. In the team setting, the insecure manager may unconsciously express negativism toward team members with whom they have a prior history. On the other hand, this same person may express unconditional support for a different team member's position, in the belief that he or she can stockpile political favors. Both behaviors reduce the manager's credibility, stifle or manipulate team members, and raise significant questions about the need for a manager on the team in the first place.

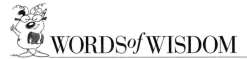

WORDS *of* WISDOM

People are never made to feel important . . . they simply are!

Assigning Work Unevenly

In the traditional bureaucracy, the assignment of desirable projects is a tool for exerting influence and rewarding others. When this reward behavior continues in the context of a team-based organization, the selection of a "chosen few" or a "team within the team" results. The remaining team members lose interest and commitment. Distrust, defensiveness, reduced commitments, unnecessary conflicts, turnover in team members, attendance problems, and resentment about having to do their work are red flags. Their presence suggests that team productivity is or will soon be seriously compromised by unfair reward practices. *It is a leadership imperative* to make sure people are not overlooked for involvement, that the team has adequate resources, and that teams are formally recognized for their efforts, even in the face of mistakes.

STRATEGIES TO CORRECT SELF-ESTEEM ISSUES IN TEAMS

Be Tactful in the Manner Applied to Check for Accuracy

Regularly ask for feedback and aim for diplomacy. "Can you help me understand how you reached that conclusion?" "Can you tell me more about this?" Use your facial expressions and beckoning hand gestures to indicate that you truly *do* want to understand. One of the most fatal flaws of managers is an abrasive, intimidating, or bullying style, which reflects a habitual insensitivity to others.

Provide the Opportunity for Team Members to Express Their Own Expertise

Managers may be tempted to fill silence with talk. But silence might mean that people are thinking! Therefore managers should not be so eager to rush to action, but rather be aware of how much of the team's time is taken by listening. The manager should take the opportunity to recognize and

WORDS *of* WISDOM

When everyone has an equal opportunity to grow and contribute, there really is a great deal of control in the system ... self-control!

~

encourage crucial contradictions made by other team members and to continually ask people what they think. These actions can only build self-determination and team accountability for outcomes. When teams are asked how a problem can be solved, their capacity to handle it is developed.

Respect and Appreciate Reliability, Ingenuity, Cooperativeness, and Determination for All of the Team's Work

All work (even mistakes) takes energy, involvement, and commitment. Team members know how busy managers are. When a manager takes the time to really understand the team experience, what the team's work is, and how well (or not well) it is going, staff members are given the gift of time. This action conveys respect and support for the team more than any words could accomplish.

Never Carry a Grudge, Criticize in Front of Others, or Withhold Crucial Information

The social power of teams is developed or diminished by the supply or withholding of crucial information. Teams need information, even sensitive information, to achieve their outcomes. Managers play a key role in assisting teams to set up information systems that guarantee the right information, at the right time, in the right context. Personal feedback needs to be saved for individual interactions. Also, remember that the manager is constantly being observed by team members for the display of that behavior which is appropriate for the team setting. Grudges and criticism do not value the dignity of the human being and destroy team effectiveness.

Know Thyself Organizationally

Can you see your organization, not as it used to be, but in the context of the health care marketplace? Do you build on these observations in your

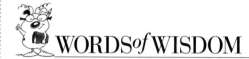

WORDS*of*WISDOM

We need to honor our teams more . . . and our dynamic leaders and radical geniuses less.

Leaders' skills are best rated not by how well systems run when they are there . . . but how well these systems work after they are gone!

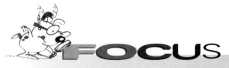

Clarifying Team Expectations

- Identify desired results.
- Facilitate team to set guidelines and parameters.
- Identify resources and access to them.
- Define accountability standards and time parameters.
- Discuss positive and negative consequences of action and nonaction.

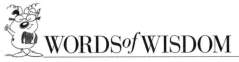

WORDS of WISDOM

Lightning only strikes in one place because that place is not there any longer!

~

role as teacher-in-chief in your organization? Do you have a clear perception of where your organization is headed?

Leaders' main tasks are to energize their organizations and to display a consistent willingness to act. This means knowing how, why, and when organizational structures, processes, and systems *prevent* action!

Encourage Self-Observation and Self-Evaluation through Modeling, Active Listening, and Feedback to the Team*

These behaviors encourage teams to ask for and gather the resources they need for success, as well as in the setting of appropriate performance goals.

Encourage Self-Reinforcement and Self-Expectations†

Expectation setting and reinforcement processes assist the team to generate those team controls which will have a direct impact on performance. The most effective control systems are knowledge induced, are backed by data-driven decisions, and are self-induced.

Encourage Rehearsal So That a Team Practices an Activity Before Implementation‡

This activity allows the team to validate their action plan, anticipate obstacles, and modify actions if necessary. This meaningful work is sometimes overlooked in well-functioning teams but is just as important. Avoid the mistake of dodging rehearsal because it feels contrived or uncomfortable. As they practice, people learn how to perform in the context of a team. The information gained is well worth the effort.

---

*Manz CC, Sims HP: Leading workers to lead themselves. The external leadership of self-managing teams, *Administrative Science Quarterly* 32(1): 106-128, 1987.
†Manz CC: Self-leadership: toward an expanded theory of self-influence processes in organizations, *Academy of Management Review* 11(13): 585-600, 1994.
‡Cohen SG et al: A predictive model of self-managing work team effectiveness, *Human Relations* 49(5): 643-677, 1996.

Foster Self-Regulation

It is tempting to direct poorly performing teams, but such interventions interfere with the development of self-regulation. In fact, Beekun (1989) found that some self-managing teams perform better *without managers*. It cannot be overemphasized that managers must leave behind their supervisory persona when interacting with teams and replace outdated behaviors with team facilitation skills, or their contributions will soon be deemed unnecessary.

WHAT DO YOU BELIEVE ABOUT LEADERSHIP?

What you believe about leadership drives your behaviors and is influenced by the general values and issues of your formative work life period. What are your own leadership metaphors? When you describe leadership in organizations, are leaders the head of the living organism? Or do you believe that wisdom is distributed throughout the system in an integrated, holistic, and natural manner?

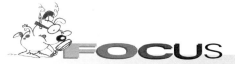

What Do You Believe about the Work of Health Care?

- Do you have no doubt that more and more health care work is knowledge-based rather than industrial, creating new demands on the labor force?
- Can you give credence to observations that health care services are no longer a consultation of individual services, but the result of an aggregate of cross-functional, interdependent performance arrangements?
- Do you believe that leadership in the new organization will pass from person-to-person or from team-to-team? Do you believe that people will come and go as new needs surface?

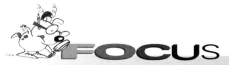

What Do You Believe about Leadership and Change?

- Do you believe that change forces people to create new ways of being and doing?
- Do you accept the notion that change makes it possible for organizations to keep up with rapid changes in service and economic demands?
- Do you recognize that, in your own organization, people's access to improved information systems results in all changes (once felt only locally) being experienced everywhere in the organization at the same time?
- Can you accept that to be an authentic change agent means being willing to risk everything (even your job, if necessary) to accomplish the objectives of change?

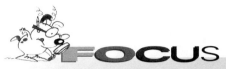

Leadership must be the part of every project team, by managers who stimulate questioning, team self-management capability, and readiness to act. Formal leaders are freed to meet their accountability for integrating, resourcing, and orchestrating the complex interaction of systems, within the context of the business and service responsibility. Teams are not an end unto themselves, but a means to achieve the organizational goals of quality and service, in the context of enhanced productivity.

DYSFUNCTIONAL ROLE ADAPTATIONS

Why do some managers fail while others grow to new levels of vitality? In leadership positions, when the leader's self-esteem is low, we see the twin symptoms of self-doubt and false pride, and an unfailing, consistent practice of viewing others through a negative filter (Blanchard, 1996). When negative perceptions of others persist, manager behaviors become threats to, rather than drivers of, team productivity.

Two dysfunctional manager role adaptations are developing in today's changing organizations. They contribute to the eventual failure of individuals in meeting new manager role demands: the self-doubting leader and the warrior leader (Blanchard, 1996).

The Self-Doubting Leader

Today's health care manager is struggling with uncertainty because the foundations of management practice have been shaken to the core. The recognition that what has always worked in the past no longer produces successful outcomes is at best unsettling and at worst paralyzing. To make matters worse, even if managers do produce good outcomes, circumstances may produce job loss anyway. When managers fail to take a true accounting of their own strengths and weaknesses and do not act on them, the outcome can be a dysfunctional role adaptation described as the *self-doubting leader* (Box 6-1). These individuals may find themselves at even greater career risk because organizations no longer have safe harbors, or "parking places," for risk-averse leaders.

The Warrior Leader

On the other end of the continuum are managers who have a high need for power and control. They love to make war. However, the *warrior leader* is also a dysfunctional role adaptation to manager self-esteem deficits (Box 6-2). This style masks competence fears with arrogance and pseudo-risk taking behaviors. The language of the warrior manager includes references to "war chests," "preparing to do battle," "winning or losing," and "taking on the enemy." In reality, the warrior manager's actions are dictated by a certain false pride, stemming from a lack of self-esteem and an underdeveloped set of core values. If unchecked, these managers temporarily boost their own low self-esteem by taking away the self-esteem of others.

WHERE ARE YOU IN YOUR OWN TRANSFORMATION?

When leaders come from a position of self-esteem, their actions and the quality of their relationships are positive. Positive relationships create positive results! These leaders can hear feedback, corral the compulsion to act prematurely, and accept criticism and praise without suspecting manipula-

BOX 6-1

Are You or Someone You Know a Self-Doubting Leader?

- Do you dodge or postpone difficult decisions?
- Do you find yourself avoiding conflict?
- Are you described as never around and not very helpful?
- Are you easily influenced by the last person who spoke to you?
- Do you rarely rock the boat?
- Do you fail to support your people when the stakes are high?
- In times of drastic change, do you seek excuses for nonaction?
- Do you find yourself listening to the 10% of folks who resist change?

BOX 6-2

Are You or Someone You Know a Warrior Manager?

- Do you fail to support your people because of your high degree of self-interest?
- Are you usually suspicious of other peoples' real motives?
- Even when it is clear that you are wrong, do you boast that you are right?
- Do you support only those who will help you move up the next step in the hierarchy?
- Do you engage in behavior that for anyone else would be judged arrogant?
- Do you believe that you are immune from the judgments applied to others?

Most of what we call management today consists of making it difficult for people to do their jobs.

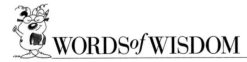

WORDS *of* WISDOM

What counts is what you learn after you know it all!

~

tion. Praise is easy to give to others because it is not perceived as taking anything away from oneself. When employees must be counseled, it is done in a manner that respects the dignity and worth of the person. People receive the direction and coaching that they need. Difficult decisions are enacted rather than avoided, and the contributions of others are acknowledged. Evolution requires something to deteriorate for something new to come alive. A manager can be viewed as a sort of fertilizer, food for the living energy present in organizations, as well as those who follow in the manager's footsteps.

A little honor of the self can go a long way for today's manager. Honor translates into responsible behavior, expressing a genuine way to care for those served: patients and staff members. One way to honor oneself is to engage in a purposeful self-examination of one's managerial strengths and weaknesses. This form of self-care is intimately tied to self-esteem because it implies self-importance: what a manager does is important, and the manager's impact on others is important. Whether formally educated in business principles or educated on the job, the manager's self-evaluation must include the leadership factors discussed in this chapter: quality of work relationships, beliefs about leadership, and operational strengths and weaknesses.

MOVING TOWARD KARIOS

The Greek poet Hesiod wrote about turning points in human life-moments called *karios*, which means a moment of transformation or metamorphosis, after which nothing is the same. We all have these touchstone moments of truth, when insights are gained and truth becomes manifest.

Managers responsible for realigning organizational structures from hierarchy and department-based models to point-of-service and team-based arrangements have their own experience of karios, when they experience flashes of insight about themselves and their own practices. Finding oneself confronted with the truth about outdated organizational behaviors enables one to address the real obstacles to team-based managerial practices.

Turning Points

Consider these insights, discovered and now acted on by contemporary managers who are successfully practicing in team-based systems:

1. In a team-based organization, knowledge once monopolized by managers must now be redistributed to assist those working at the point-of-service (Blanchard, 1996). *Power realized through information will no longer be an effective manager behavior.*

2. The right to know is a basic truth. Rather than focusing on what is safe to say at any point in time, it is better to err on sharing too much (Drucker, 1985). *I will no longer control information flow, and this will cause me great anxiety at times.*

3. Hoarded information is pointless power. *If I continue to hoard information, my teams will not achieve their outcomes.*

4. Even when we get everyone in the same room and make sure that they have the same information, there will be different levels of commitment. *I will have to understand more about how people in teams work and grow in different ways. People need different things from me.*

5. An individual without information can remain confused, while a person with the right information must be accountable. Goals and objectives do not establish a foundation for accountability; coaching, teaching, learning, and information do. *These must be the cornerstones of my management practices.*

6. Hierarchy demands that managers be parents and that workers be children. Fearing punishment for mistakes, workers delegate responsibility upward. *I must unlearn the psychology of control that has served me in the past.*

7. New work relationships require relationships of reciprocity, where each person takes responsibility within a framework of ground rules that can be changed to improve performance (Toffler, 1990). *I will discard those partial truths that keep me operating as a human machine who controls people.*

WHERE ARE YOU?

VICTIM
- Why should I bother?
- I just go with the flow.
- It's hopeless.

PASSIVE EMPOWERMENT
- I'm waiting for the next promotion.
- If I am patient my day will come.

ACTIVE EMPOWERMENT
- I can make a difference.
- I take initiative and use my influence.

HIGHLY ACTIVE EMPOWERMENT
- I am committed to influence the organization, people, and events.
- I take balanced risks.
- I use my position description as a guide, not a constraint.

8. No matter how long you have been working under a particular set of assumptions, a day for change comes. *Power does not welcome change. I can no longer participate in organizational rituals that punish innovation and dissent.*

9. Participation is not something that the top orders the middle to do for the bottom (Toffler, 1990). *When I treat participation as a luxury, it is an insult to those I lead.*

10. To empower people in unaligned organizations is counterproductive. I alone cannot create the conditions for empowerment. *I must work with other leaders in my organization and purposefully redistribute power at the point-of-service . . . where the service really occurs.*

11. We must get away from the dualistic, destructive thinking in which there is one and then there is the other. *To build team-based systems, I must be able to see that there is not the other, but only the one—the whole.*

12. No matter how much effort you put into something or how much you prepare, you will make mistakes. *If I want to succeed, I must double my failure rate* (Maccoby, 1993).

Sometimes people prefer to avoid the more unpleasant pieces of their work. However, real transformation will occur only if we struggle to identify who we really are as managers. This requires uncovering and recognizing the full impact of our leadership actions, as well as truthfully examining all the dimensions of our organization. Without soul searching, managers can fall victim to change rather than lead it.

BEFORE MOVING TO A TEAM-BASED SYSTEM

Strong leaders understand human behavior. To move into a team-based system is not a small decision. Certain factors must be carefully examined so that planning and implementation activities change behavior.

One of the most challenging factors associated with this type of change is assisting employees to become comfortable with the ambiguity of a newly reorganized workplace. At times, it is not clear what if any benefits result from the change. For the staff members and middle managers, real-

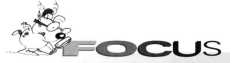

FOCUS

Twelve Moments of Truth

1. *Power realized through information will no longer be an effective behavior.*
2. *I will no longer control information flow, and this will cause me great anxiety.*
3. *If I continue to hoard information, my teams will not achieve their outcomes.*
4. *I will have to understand more about how people in teams work and grow in different ways. People need different things from me.*
5. *Coaching, teaching, learning, and information must be the cornerstones of my management practices.*
6. *I must unlearn the psychology of control that has served me in the past.*
7. *I will discard those partial truths that keep me operating as a human machine who controls people.*
8. *Power does not welcome change. I can no longer participate in organizational rituals that punish innovation and dissent.*
9. *When I treat participation as a luxury, it is an insult to those I lead.*
10. *I must work with other leaders in my organization and purposefully redistribute power at the point-of-service . . . where the service really occurs.*
11. *To build team-based systems, I must be able to see that there is not the other, but only the one-the whole.*
12. *If I want to succeed, I must double my failure rate.*

ity is the harshest at these ambiguous points in time, because they usually did not have a role in making the decision to move to a team-based system. Managing change is managing relationships. Without effective organizational preparation, the complex transition to teams will be fraught with stumbling blocks, regardless of how detailed the planning process is.

Sometimes teams have been implemented in a hierarchical structure under the guise of quality improvement. However, these teams have no real organizational authority for action and become nothing more than busywork that is disliked by everyone.

People are organized into teams, and "teamtalk" is prevalent in the organization. However, parallel management structures, such as the operations meeting, continue to be the real decision-making structures for the organization. No one addresses actually making the teams work, and thus they eventually disband.

Consider the experience of one health care organization, where disease management rounds were instituted with a multidisciplinary staff. Format and tools were created, and the momentum for the change was high. However, planning did not accurately accommodate physician preparation for involvement. Consequently, doctors verbally supported the program but failed to attend rounds. Disease management plans were delayed, physicians were labeled as resistors, and staff members lost their initial enthusiasm. Organizational preparation for the change had failed to address physician expectations for the disease management program and the behavioral changes that would be required for the physician's successful participation.

Reorganizing people into effective team structures must be accompanied by a prepared and focused management team. Management must address several critical questions before pursuing the complex work of developing people who have the capacity for self-management, accountability, and teamwork:

1. Can all managers accept the fact that authority and accountability will no longer be the exclusive domain of management, but will be shared by all employees?

2. How effective is your communication system? In preparation for change, conduct an audit of every piece of communication. Is it cross-functional? Check for consistency and stakeholder needs and gaps.

3. How will you maintain functional expertise in your teams? The everyday nature of work, including vacations, transfers, and absences, will require "in-between" solutions. You must ensure that technical pools or outsourcing decisions will be congruent with the organization's financial goals for them to be supported in real-time implementation.

What will remain vertical and what will be horizontally aligned in teams? Strategy and finance usually remain vertical. Human resources (HR) has been made both vertical and horizontal, with HR support assigned to each service pathway. Utilization management and discharge planning have been combined into case management and horizontally integrated into teams.

Bibliography

Beekun RI: Assessing the effectiveness of sociotechnical interventions: antidote or fad? *Human Relations* 42(7):877-897, 1989.

Blanchard K: Self-esteem and the management of others. In Canfield J, Miller J (eds): *Heart at work,* New York, McGraw-Hill, 1996.

Bridges W: Leading the de-jobbed organization. In Hesselbein F, Goldsmith M, Beckhard R (eds): *The leader of the future,* San Francisco, Jossey-Bass, 1996.

Cohen SG, Ladford GE, Speitzler GM: A predictive model of self-managing work team effectiveness, *Human Relations* 49(5):643-677, 1996.

Cyr R: Maintaining employee self-esteem, *Supervisory Management* 37(6):1-3, 1992.

Drucker P: *The changing world of the executive,* New York, Times Books, 1985.

Kanter RM: *The change masters,* New York, Simon and Schuster, 1986.

Kriegel R, Brandt D: *Sacred cows make the best burgers,* New York, Warner Books, 1996.

Maccoby M: Managers must unlearn the psychology of control, *Research Technology Management* (25):2, 49-51, 1993.

Manz CC: Self-leadership: toward an expanded theory of self-influence processes in organizations, *Academy of Management Review* 11(13):585-600, 1994.

Manz CC, Sims HP: Leading workers to lead themselves. The external leadership of self-managing teams, *Administrative Science Quarterly* 32(1):106-128, 1987.

Oshry B: *Seeing systems,* San Francisco, Berrett-Koehler, 1995.

Schor JB: *The overworked American,* New York, Basic Books, 1992.

Toffler A: *Powershift: knowledge, wealth and violence at the edge of the 21st century,* New York, Bantam Books, 1990.

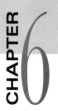

TOOLCHEST

TOOL A: Customized Self-Improvement Matrix

Instructions: Using the self-improvement matrix grid (Table 6-1), think about each of the operational activities listed and your degree of confidence in performing that function, as well as how much you enjoy doing that particular type of work. Consider the following questions as you perform that function to help complete the matrix grid.

- Do you perform it with more or less reflex? Is there more or less thought put into your actions?
- How often do you find yourself engaging in blame or confusion when performing the function?
- How compassionate are you when doing the work?
- How empowered do you feel when functioning in this performance area?

- On a scale of 1 to 5, with 5 being a high lack of confidence and a least enjoyable part of your work as a manager, circle your feelings about each performance area.

Once you have completed the questionnaire, look back over your performance areas to identify which areas may be sources of self-doubt. Scores of 4 or 5 suggest challenges to self-confidence in performing the function. It is here that you want to set targets for performance improvement. *Hint:* This tool can also be used to develop a self-directed work team or in a team-building session with managers, to receive feedback on their performance from others.

TABLE **6-1**

Self-Improvement Matrix					
PERFOMANCE AREA	**LACK CONFIDENCE**	**LEAST ENJOY**	**PERFORMANCE AREA**	**LACK CONFIDENCE**	**LEAST ENJOY**
Resource Management			Reducing resources	1 2 3 4 5	1 2 3 4 5
Staffing	1 2 3 4 5	1 2 3 4 5	Leadership	1 2 3 4 5	1 2 3 4 5
Variance analysis	1 2 3 4 5	1 2 3 4 5	Organizational influence	1 2 3 4 5	1 2 3 4 5
Statistics	1 2 3 4 5	1 2 3 4 5	Department/unit influence	1 2 3 4 5	1 2 3 4 5
Recordkeeping	1 2 3 4 5	1 2 3 4 5	Vision setting	1 2 3 4 5	1 2 3 4 5
Materials management	1 2 3 4 5	1 2 3 4 5	My behavior congruence	1 2 3 4 5	1 2 3 4 5

TABLE **6-1**, *cont'd*

Self-Improvement Matrix

PERFOMANCE AREA	LACK CONFIDENCE	LEAST ENJOY	PERFORMANCE AREA	LACK CONFIDENCE	LEAST ENJOY
Resource Management, *cont'd*			**Systems**		
Time management	1 2 3 4 5	1 2 3 4 5	Integration of information technology	1 2 3 4 5	1 2 3 4 5
Tight deadlines	1 2 3 4 5	1 2 3 4 5	Building interdisciplinary operation	1 2 3 4 5	1 2 3 4 5
Priority setting	1 2 3 4 5	1 2 3 4 5	Constructing a continuum of care	1 2 3 4 5	1 2 3 4 5
Fiscal Management			Seeing patterns	1 2 3 4 5	1 2 3 4 5
Business planning	1 2 3 4 5	1 2 3 4 5	Making networks	1 2 3 4 5	1 2 3 4 5
Marketing	1 2 3 4 5	1 2 3 4 5	Building and maintaining management systems	1 2 3 4 5	1 2 3 4 5
Resource allocation	1 2 3 4 5	1 2 3 4 5			
Program development	1 2 3 4 5	1 2 3 4 5	**Relationships**		
Support			Superior	1 2 3 4 5	1 2 3 4 5
Team outcome achievement	1 2 3 4 5	1 2 3 4 5	Colleague	1 2 3 4 5	1 2 3 4 5
Staff empowerment and decision relocation	1 2 3 4 5	1 2 3 4 5	Board of trustees	1 2 3 4 5	1 2 3 4 5
Conflict mediation	1 2 3 4 5	1 2 3 4 5	Staff	1 2 3 4 5	1 2 3 4 5
Performance appraisal	1 2 3 4 5	1 2 3 4 5			
Values clarification	1 2 3 4 5	1 2 3 4 5			
Teaching/mentoring	1 2 3 4 5	1 2 3 4 5			
Team building	1 2 3 4 5	1 2 3 4 5			

Scoring Instructions

Add the scores for each item and compare your self-improvement matrix with the ratings below.

0-40   Evaluate yourself again. This score means you are extremely self-confident. Are you sure there are no areas for improvement?

41-80   You are confident about most aspects of your work. Examine items in which you scored yourself 4 or 5 and create a plan for improvement.

81-120 You have a mixed review of your own performance. Focus on the items scored at 4 or 5 and get support in improving your performance.

121-160 You are struggling with several aspects of your management position. If you are to remain in management you must act now to correct performance issues.

161-200 Scores at this level suggest that you do not feel prepared to operate in a management position. Reconsider your fit with a managerial role or pursue an aggressive action plan to build your management skills.

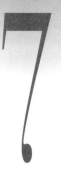

Supporting Teams: Creating Seamless Linkage

A process and its related work is only as effective as the structures which sustain it.

Porter-O'Grady

The locus of control for decisions moves to the point-of-service, which requires the structure for decision making to move closer to where the work is done. This affects the control and power distribution in the system.

Teams require a different organizational configuration to be sustainable. Using the same organizational structure as applied to departments will simply not work for teams.

NEW WAYS OF MAKING DECISIONS TOGETHER

Team-based decisions assume an operating infrastructure makes it possible for teams to operate effectively. The problem in most organizations is that such an infrastructure is not truly present.

The move from individual departmental, vertically oriented structures to horizontal interdisciplinary, integrated systems requires a tremendous shift in the foundation for supporting the decision making that occurs in these environments. Furthermore, linking the decisions of one group to another, and ensuring that the flow of decisions and information generated by those decisions is available to all whom the decisions affect, is a major consideration for the organization. The challenges are significant:

- People do not know how to link their individual decisions with those of the team.
- The team is such a new concept for work that linking teams' work with each other is also challenging for the system.

- Individuals have not developed a strong enough relationship with each other within a team context to know just what communication and decision-making processes are individual and what are collective.
- Whatever system supports exist, they are generated essentially by the manager; the kind of information the manager historically has received is no longer appropriate to the kind of information that the team needs to sustain itself.
- Much of the orientation of the system is to vertical decision making initiated predominantly by managers. Increasingly, decisions must be initiated by team members, which changes the locus of control for decision making in the organization.
- Staff members, while generally good at making individual decisions, are not necessarily expert at making collective decisions and conscientiously acknowledging the processes associated with decision making. Teaching these processes and making them the modus operandi of the organization will be a major challenge for leadership.
- The organization is not familiar with allowing decisions to generate in places other than the management frame of reference. Top-down decision making is a generally acceptable method for decision making. The "point-of-service outward" decision process is a relatively new approach to decision making. This shift in decision making accountability creates a challenge in the role of the manager and shifts the obligation of that role into other arenas for which the manager may not be adequately prepared.

Each of these challenges brings a host of activities necessary to address their implications into the process of team-based development for the organization. Each of these issues will have a major impact on the effectiveness of the organization in making team-based decisions and creating a relationship between and among teams and team members. Any constraints must be addressed in some formal way as the organizational structure unfolds to support team-based decision-making processes.

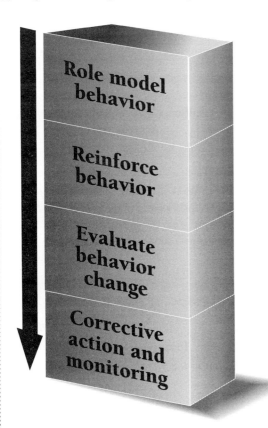

Fewer managers in health systems are needed as the systems become more decentralized. However, there is an increasing requirement for competence and effectiveness in the manager. Skill development is the most important activity of managers in the new team-based organization.

BOX 7-1

Moving decisions to the point-of-service requires a change in the role of the manager:
- Develop staff members' skills in decision making
- Support staff members in making decisions
- Use problems as tools for skill building
- Let go of parenting role with the staff
- Gather information for staff as required by decisions
- Evaluate effectiveness of decision processes of staff
- Undertake corrective action as early as possible
- Guide staff in understanding political content of decisions
- Help staff celebrate small successes

Change does not occur in a straight line. It cycles around, sometimes repeating what once was and immediately following that with a new frame of reference that challenges thinking and doing. Change feels more schizophrenic than it fluid.

CHANGE IN THE ROLE EXPECTATIONS FOR THE MANAGER

Team-based decision making changes the role of manager in radical ways, as outlined in earlier chapters. However, what is critical to understanding the change in the role of the manager and its functional impact on decision making is the need to define specific arenas in which the manager has accountability (Box 7-1). The manager also needs to know those areas of decision making for which she or he does not have accountability. Many academics and management theorists would suggest that such clear differentiation is not a necessary undertaking for the organization, that much of this will flow as the developmental processes toward team mature. It has, however, been the author's experience that this does not occur in such fluid ways because most change appears, on the surface at least, schizophrenic and incremental. So also does the developmental processes around a change in the locus of control, authority, and decision making in the organization. What facilitates this shift is a clear delineation of those areas of performance expectation that are differentiated from those that have always been present. This means clearly defining in advance what some of those expectations are, even if those expectations shift over time. Defining them at the outset gives a clear indication to all players of a significant shift in the organization's emphasis and a change in the expectations for behavior and decision making.

The manager, perhaps, has the most significant amount of work to do in making change happen. Two specific issues confront the manager in her or his shift to new roles. The first issue relates to the manager's own behaviors, expectations, and role shifts. The second relates to the manager's obligation to see that those same behaviors and role shift changes occur in the behaviors of staff members and teams. Much of the decision making that was once a part of the manager's role now must become a part of the team's role. The manager must not only be willing to become unattached to decisions that she or he once owned, but facilitate the development of the skills necessary to exercise those decisions in others who now have the obligation for them.

The manager, furthermore, has additional obligations to ensure that successful outcomes are achieved. One of the most significant shifts to horizontal and team-based organizations is the role the manager has in ensuring that the decisions made by teams and staff members are carried out as anticipated. When this does not occur or is compromised, those issues are laid on the table, dealt with, clarified, and resolved by those who own them.

Much of the change of the manager's role is from direction to facilitation, from telling to mentoring, from parenting to participation, from focus on process to emphasis on outcome. Each of these changes has an elemental impact on the role of the manager and the skill base necessary to operate in the new frame of reference. This skill base and new set of expectations creates challenges for the manager that will have to be dealt with specifically (see Chapter 4). This twofold challenge, a shift in the manager's behavior and an expectation of developing staff to make effective decisions, creates a tremendous burden on the manager's role in the decision-making process.

In team-based structures, there is a need for fewer managers. Increasingly, it is evident that an inverse relationship exists between the number of managers in a system and its effectiveness and efficiency. The outcomes associated with this emerging mindset require that more effectiveness and efficient management decision making occur closer to the point-of-service as fewer managers exist in the system. In all team-based approaches, because decision making is made at the point-of-service and is predominantly based within the team framework, the number and variety of managers in the system who take the burden for making decisions for staff members and others are not present. Therefore the removal of the manager creates conditions necessary to deal with issues that she or he once dealt with, insulated the staff from, and resolved outside the cycle of team-based decision making. This challenge means that the issues themselves are presented to the staff members with no intervening resolution by a third party, notably the man-

Although it is difficult to accept, there is a need for fewer managers in organizations than in the past. Managers and staff members must be aware that team-based approaches require more accountability at the staff level, and this will ultimately change both the numbers and roles of managers in the system.

Staff members are not fully capable of making team-based decisions simply because they are now members of teams. The organization must provide a learning process for team members that helps with the transition. Without this, organizational leaders should not expect to have effective teams or good decisions in their system.

CHANGE IN DECISION STRUCTURES

Industrial age

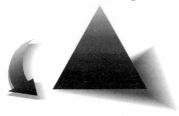

Transitional matrix

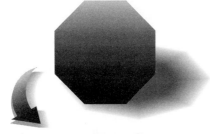

New organizational decision format

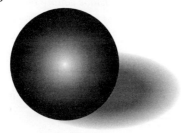

Creating a team-based system is a learning process. All members of the system are learners. The manager must represent in her or his behavior a commitment to learning, growing, and modeling that to others.

ager of the past. The manager in a team-based system not only has the obligation to change the focus of decision making but, to survive, she or he *must* change that focus. The manager has additional obligations to see that those decisions are made effectively and that the organization is not compromised during the transition period between the old management system and the new team-based system. There is clearly a developmental and learning cycle in the organization during which time a high risk exists for decisions not being made or not being effective and perhaps even being inadequate and inappropriate. The challenge for the manager is a continuing awareness of the possibility of such circumstances and the need to put in place some transitional processes that assist her or him in making decisions as needed and facilitating decision making in the staff. At the beginning of change to team-based decision making, the manager would make more decisions. As the team matures, the skill base develops, and the shift of locus of control continues, the manager's expectation would be to make fewer decisions and to see that more of them are made within the team context.

ISSUES WITH TEAM-BASED DECISION MAKING

Simply because staff members should be involved in decision making does not guarantee that they have the skills necessary to do so. Staff members come out of the traditional organizational system where ownership for decisions rest with the organization and follow the management track. Issues in that frame of reference create demands on the staff that result in frustration, anger, and sometimes questioning the appropriateness of such a shift. Staff members already feel overburdened with the amount of obligation and energy they must commit to work. Increasing that burden with the expectation that they be involved in more broad-based decision making that affects how the team works, its resources, issues of applying the team process, outcome determination, and evaluation processes do not encourage interest in the team-based developmental process. Clearly, in staff members' minds there is additional work involved.

The truth is that at the outset, there is additional work. The problem at the transitional phase toward teams is the conflict between old expectations and new requirements of team members. What individuals often fail to recognize is that it is not simply doing more with less that is critical, it is actually doing differently in the organization that creates the strongest commitment on the part of the staff.

Staff members frequently attempt to continue to work as they have in the past, but with fewer resources, limited time, and less external support. This is not possible in the new frame of reference. What must be communicated to the staff is that the design, structuring, and implementation of new models of service require that organization to be different and perform its work in different ways. There must be a different emphasis in terms of what the work is. There should be a clear expectation on the part of the clinical leaders to identify new frames of reference for work, processes that indicate what is effective and noneffective, and evaluation mechanisms that delineate which activities are appropriate and which are not. All of this requires a different mindset on the part of staff members.

INCREASING STAFF MEMBER INVOLVEMENT ON TEAMS

Clearly, the organizational noise associated with this shift is considerable. The demands in creating a new frame of reference for staff-based decision making and the behaviors that it represents requires different kinds of organizational supports from the system as well. Simply changing the system and requiring that the staff do differently is not a sufficient demand on the part of the system. Often one of the most traumatic experiences in unfolding changing care structures or reengineered systems is that the supporting infrastructure and the organizational supports to the staff necessary to make meaningful change and to operate within a new milieu are not present. Therefore staff members move into a new organizational model and new patient care decision-making structures, only to find that they do not have the necessary supporting structure, informational infrastructure, position investment, and organizational resources to be successful.

In the new organization staff members cannot expect to see that their needs are taken care of by the organization. No system can protect everyone from the vagaries of change. To thrive the system must always change. If a staff member is not adaptable to the change there is likely a problem with "fit" between that person and system. The only way to resolve this issue is to become involved or to leave.

153

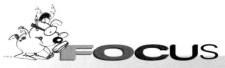

Continuous development means:
- *Everyone in the organization partici-pates in learning (including doctors and administrators), no exceptions.*
- *Goals for learning are defined by the organization, teams, and individuals, ensuring that all are "singing off the same song sheet."*
- *Leaders (both managers and clini-cians) gather regularly to assess progress and to encourage each other's work in advancing and ful-filling the work and vision of the system.*

No team-based processes can last long without a supporting infrastructure that brings form to the team, champions its work, and invests in the members of the team.

Therefore, as patient care staff members struggle to meet the needs of those they serve or accommodate the changes in the organizational system while operating with fewer resources, they become less and less able to meet the demands of their work. The context or the milieu within which they operate is not sufficiently supporting the activities they are obligated to address. Staff members, as a result, become overwhelmed, angry, and re-actionary with the whole notion and idea associated with a reengineered organizational system.

In this chapter we focus on three specific components of the decision-making infrastructure that are necessary to ensure that team-based and in-tegrated care models operate successfully. This infrastructure is a critical component of creating a seamless and continuous decision-making frame-work for the organizational system and requires commitment of the re-sources of the organization necessary to build the infrastructure support-ing team-based decision making. Without this infrastructure there is con-siderable challenge to the success of any attempt to build team-based approaches to decision making. The three supporting structures are: a con-tinuous learning system, an information infrastructure, and a clinical model for service delivery.

A CONTINUOUS LEARNING SYSTEM

A continuous learning system is not simply team building. While much fo-cus is on the process of team building, the system that supports it reflects an entirely different characterization of a system and its fundamental re-sponsibilities to both the organization that makes it up and the people it serves. A learning system focuses on continuous development as a funda-mental functional part of the organizational construct. Indeed it is assumed that such development is an integral part of the obligation of the system to the work that it does. Resources, therefore, are devoted specifically and di-rectly to addressing the issues of continuing development and growth as a part of the work of the organization.

In the "old" organization education was looked at as a requisite of the system, but generally identified as an extra component that the system committed to facilitate the growth of its staff and the quality of its work. Although that was a valid and viable approach to the learning process for many organizations, it is no longer adequate at a time of great change. Adjustment in both the focus of service and the character of health care delivery is required as it goes through a major transformation. At least during the transformative process, but likely during the life of service, commitment to learning as an ongoing part of the organization's construct is an important consideration to the design and structuring of organizational systems.

The Department of Education

In the old model, education was looked at much like the other components of the organization's structure, as a compartmentalized functional activity that had its own characteristics, obligations, and expectations. In the new organizational system the approach to education from a departmental perspective is no longer adequate. The locus of education within a departmental framework means that the obligation the organization sees for education is also departmentalized or externalized from that obligation each individual has to his or her own learning and development. What it assumes is that education or learning is a functional component of the organization rather than an operational expectation of the system.

In the old model of education, department educators were hired whose purpose was to transfer information and to see that appropriate education and skill development occurred in the various components of the organization that needed it. Furthermore, the more general requirements that came from the accrediting bodies or the regulatory agencies were also included in the expectation for education that educators would bring to the organization. Fundamentally, education was considered the work of this department, and the obligation of the providers was to bring education to the organization and its individuals as the demand required. Education was looked at as an external and functional activity of the organization.

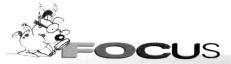

FOCUS

Being able to deal with the "noise" of personal change is critical to thriving in the chaos of change. Individuals must learn to listen to themselves:
- *Feelings of tension require some means of expression through verbalizing and physical expression—never keep it "in" or quiet.*
- *Get together with colleagues and find ways of expression and support for each other—often.*
- *Never let a problem with another fester. It does not shrink with time. Expressing the concern safely and positively addresses both the issue and the relationship.*

No more departments. The basic unit of work is the team. All work will be configured around the patient in partnerships between providers at the point-of-service.

Teams define learning needs specific to the needs of the team.

Teams define a program of learning for their members.

Teams evaluate the impact of learning on their work and adjust performance.

Learning is a lifelong experience necessary to advance any career. A worker is at high risk today if his or her learning activities have ended.

Team-Driven Education

In the new frame of reference, where the locus of control is at the point-of-service, where decision making unfolds within the context of the staff, and the organization's focus and emphasis as well as structural supports is on the point-of-service, the whole process of education must be revisited. Clearly, the locus of control is no longer identified within a departmental structure. Much of the issues and decisions that relate to competence, effectiveness, skill base, and all of the other elements of efficiency and effectiveness in the organizational system are now located within the context of the team at the point-of-service.

Learning in this set of circumstances can no longer be considered an externally directed exercise. Individuals from outside the circle of obligation or the point-of-service can no longer expect to come within the point-of-service and provide what education and learning would be necessary there on an ongoing basis. The external orientation, the locus of control that emphasizes a more functional frame of reference for learning, can no longer be assumed as an appropriate model for the learning process. The ownership for learning and the obligation to make decisions related to it also belong within the cycle of decision making at the point-of-service.

Furthermore, in the team-based approach the system resources, support structures, and expectations emphasize control and decision making within the context of the team. Therefore it is expected that ownership of decisions, obligation for investment, and commitment to those decisions also exist within the context of the team. If this frame of reference is the expectation for function and activity in the organization it is also the demand for learning and development. Most learning and development must reflect the needs that emerge at the point-of-service for differentiated practice environments, integrated delivery of service, a different framework for building the continuum of care, and a changing skill base to effectively manage care delivery in that framework. Clearly, control must also exist at that point-of-service.

A Shift in Learning Framework

The organization has an increasing obligation for the design of the learning environment not only in relationship to structuring learning but the planning processes associated with development and learning around team-based approaches. This is not simply teaching people how to behave in teams and developing the teams. It is building a model of learning that requires a commitment at the point-of-service to a learning agenda moderated on the needs of individuals at the point-of-service and a continuing dynamic that raises the standard of expectation and ultimately improves the outcomes of care. This model of learning should thread throughout the organizational system to create a framework for the learning process that represents the team-based focus of the organization yet ties learning into the expectations for service outcomes enumerated in the mission and strat-

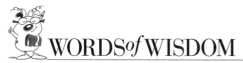

WORDS*of* WISDOM

The organization should never take away the obligation for one's own learning and career management from the staff. In order to deal with the staff in an adult-to-adult interchange, it is important for the staff to be in charge of their own partnership with the organization.

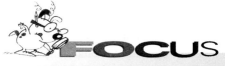

FOCUS

All learners are unit based. It is advisable that all teaching-learning activities be included there for several reasons:

1. *In an adult environment, learners do best when applying learning immediately.*
2. *Most of learning is an experiential process and requires that it be useful.*
3. *The learner should also be the teacher.*
4. *Individuals are responsible for their own learning.*
5. *Learning should be directed to helping the learners achieve a specific set of goals.*
6. *Learning must have some value and make a difference in how the work is done.*
7. *Learning helps create more opportunities to fit the worker better to the roles that emerge in the work environment.*

TEAM**TIP**   7.1

It is always advisable to keep as much control of learning and developing within the context of the team. The team becomes the basic unit of decision making and of work. The more it is empowered to make its own decisions the better it will become at doing its work. The development of the system requires making the team as independent and as successful as possible.

egy of the organizational system. How this learning is defined and the locus of control for its development becomes critical to the future of viability of the organization as it changes its purpose and the focus of its work.

The learning plan for the organization should be as important to the structure of the system as the strategic plan (Team Tip 7-1). Indeed much of what is outlined in the strategic plan simply could not be obtained without a specified and clearly enumerated learning plan for the system. The learning plan would focus on many of the same elements that the strategic plan does because a part of its obligation is to incorporate the learning activities of the organization with the strategies that give the organization direction and meaning. The learning plan focuses on the individual activities at the point-of-service and their resonance with the organization purpose and all of the functions and activities that relate to it. Tying the learning and the strategic processes together ensures that the functional and fundamental commitment of all of the members of the system at any place in the system is directed toward those activities that fulfill the system's mission and purpose. They must translate those into meaningful and focused goals at the point-of-service. Furthermore, by defining that and engaging all players necessary to articulate the learning plan, commitment to and translation of that plan into real purposeful activity becomes a viable process with the organizational system.

CHANGING ROLES

The learning component of the organizational system now changes its focus and function from providing education to ensuring that the support systems necessary for education to occur are in place. Instead of directing and controlling the educational process it facilitates the dynamic of learning throughout the organizational system. It should tie tightly together with other human resource activities related to the development and promulgation of staff-driven activities in concert with the organization's mandates.

At the systems level it is expected that the learning leadership is involved in gathering the stakeholders in a way that facilitates the development of a broad-based learning plan consistent with the direction of the organization. This integrated multidisciplinary process associated with defining the learning plan brings players together from the various arenas and components of the organization where such a plan has value and meaning and where the organization's strategic purposes must be translated into tactics and activities at the point-of-service. Through this planning process a large framework for the system is developed out of which can be determined the specific team-based educational and learning obligations that emerge at the point-of-service.

Based on the broad-based learning plan for the organizational system, team-based learning activities can be identified specifically within the context of the team and its needs and demands in articulating and unfolding goals and activities of the team that fulfill the purposes of the organization (Box 7-2). Therefore the fit between the organization's strategy, and the tactics of the team necessary to implement them, become more clearly defined.

The locus of control for the implementation of these processes is really within the framework of the team; therefore all learning activities and developmental processes unfold within the context of the team, and leadership involved in learning activities should be located as close to the point-of-service and as near to the context of the team as possible. Planning becomes the obligation of the system as a whole. Learning becomes the obligation of each member of the team at the point-of-service. The planning activities are a systematic learning process. The implementation of learning activities is a team-based and individual set of activities. Understanding this differentiation changes the locus of control for resources directed to the developmental processes associated with learning.

The learning facilitators, coaches, or educators in this approach must be located within service pathways in direct relationship with teams. Much of the facilitation of learning, development of learning plans and approaches, and the learning process itself must unfold within the context of the team because the locus of control for implementing and applying the learning is

BOX 7-2

Team Learning

Teams will need support for the system to ensure that the tools of learning are available to team members:

- Learning tools are available on request by team members for learning purposes.
- The learning activities of the team are consistent with the learning goals of the system.
- There is a learning plan for the system and tactics to incorporate the team's learning into an overall strategy to improve the system's effectiveness.
- There are learning "coaches" available to teams to assist them in creating learning processes and evaluating whether learning has occurred.
- Each team member has a plan for learning that fits the team's goals and improves his or her contribution to the team's effectiveness, as well as advances personal skill.

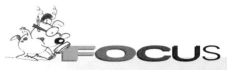

FOCUS

Creating an Individual Learning Plan

Step 1: *Think about career direction and the skill mix needs of the career. Make sure there is a good fit between career ideas and the direction of health care.*

Step 2: *Compare what you now have with regard to your career and skills and determine what learning deficit exists.*

Step 3: *Review your life choices and situation, establishing a baseline for considering what choices you will make.*

Step 4: *Make a plan of action with a step-by-step approach to getting what you need. Include a time frame.*

Step 5: *Review your plan with a mentor or someone you respect to help with finalizing your choices.*

Step 6: *Implement your plan.*

Step 7: *Continually and periodically evaluate your choices in light of current health care changes.*

at the point-of-service. Therefore the design of learning activities and processes should be incorporated at the point-of-service. Whatever educators, learning coaches, or approaches to the processes of education are used in the system, they should be located specifically and precisely at the point-of-service, where such learning has greatest value.

In the health care frame of reference roles such as clinical specialist, learning coach, educational specialist, team learning facilitator, or any other such role should be located within the service pathway at the point-of-service working directly within the context of teams and with team members. Here again, the learning process is a continuing dynamic, an expectation of the ongoing activities of work for which both time and resources should be available.

All planning on the part of the educational and learning coordinator relates specifically to the development of the team and team members. This includes activities of translating the learning plan for the system. It also specifies pathway and team-based obligations. It should articulate the model of learning and the implications of that model as applied to the learning process, identify the cultural and personal issues related to the learning process within the service pathway and each team, and identify learning activities that facilitate the advancement and effectiveness of learning process at the point-of-service.

What is perhaps the most critical role of the learning leadership at the point-of-service is the development of ownership in the staff and the team with regard to their own processes associated with learning. Because learning occurs at the point-of-service and is imbedded in the activities of unfolding the work there, the obligation and ownership for learning should also occur there. Learning should occur within the expectation that team members are a part of a learning process and have the obligation to both teach and learn. Each member of the team has a peer obligation for teaching and learning and must exemplify that in the context of his or her role. Here again, practice-based, activity-driven, point-of-service designed learning processes would include approaches not traditionally associated with the educational process in health care systems. Patient-based, case-driven, process-oriented, event-stimulated learning dynamics may be more prominent as the approaches to implementing the learning plan as formal, educational, classroom, and non-work related activities might have been in the past. Every activity in the organization serves as a foundation and framework for opportunities for learning, for advancement, and for improving the outcomes of service at the team level in the organization.

THE LEARNING COACH

One of the prominent roles emerging in new organizational structures is that of the learning coach (Box 7-3). The role of the learning coach is specifically point-of-service driven. Although the learning coach plays a major role in activities related to the learning plan, much of the functions and activities of the learning coach focus on team-based development and facilitating the viable outcomes of team-based work. The learning coach essentially is a broad-based facilitator of team activities.

In many organizations the learning coach is located within the context of each service pathway (see Chapter 2). Ostensibly, each service pathway has its own learning coach. The learning coach focuses on the following areas:

1. Assist pathway leadership in the translation of the learning plan into learning tactics and activities for the pathway and its teams.
2. Identify with the pathway leadership and team leadership the specific priorities for team development and functional enhancement to ensure effective team processes.
3. Work specifically and directly with each team in its own developmental process associated with the learning plan, its goals and activities, and its defined expectations and outcomes.
4. Work with specific teams around issues of role development and relational conflicts and issues within the context of each team's design.
5. Work specifically with team members with regard to their own developmental and relational issues with the teams or other team members. This includes conflict resolution, compatibility, and performance issues within the context of team expectations.

Much of the activities of learning require ongoing evaluation of progress. Members should stop regularly just to spend some time defining where they are and what concerns they have.

BOX **7-3**

The Learning Coach

The learning coach is a new role in organizations. This person provides the tools and format for creating the learning organization and making it live at every place its work is done. Skill development and knowledge transfer are the most important roles of this person. Her or his goal is to give away everything she or he knows to enhance the skill of others in the system.

 WORDS*of*WISDOM

Each team member is accountable for his or her own career. As we move out of the "job age," developing more fluid and mobile skill sets is important work in ensuring a personal and positive work future!

~

BOX **7-4**

The primary roles of the learning coaches
and leaders are:
1. Information transfer to team members
2. Development of good team-building
   skills
3. Development of good methods for decision making
4. Problem identification and resolution
   skill development
5. Mentor role skills as team member
6. Facilitate the development of meeting
   skills
7. Encourage leadership and risk taking
8. Push progress on planning activities
9. Evaluate progress regarding team skills
   and performance expectations
10. Identify conflict and its resolution with
    members

*Information is the life blood of any organization.
The system that handles its information well is
better positioned to thrive in this new age.*

Clearly, the learning coach has a tremendous obligation to create effective interface between the work processes of the team, the goals of the pathway, and the learning plan for the system as a whole (Box 7-4). Integrating each of these components within the activities of teams and team members creates a significant challenge to the learning coach and shifts the locus of control for learning to individuals and their teams at the point-of-service. Facilitating and focusing on this shift in the locus of control is perhaps the main obligation and benefit of a processes associated with creating a learning dynamic.

While all of these elements and activities related to a learning plan are identified in a more functional way, the underlying assumption that guides the development of learning plans and learning processes relates to all of the theoretical and organizational constructs of a learning organization. Taking learning organization theory and strategies and using them as the framework for developing both learning plans and the ownership of learning at the point-of-service becomes an important constituent of the design of effective learning as an ongoing operational element of the organizational system. Learning is looked at as a part of the dynamic of the system. Within this frame of reference all activities in the system have imbedded within them components of a learning dynamic and process that is fundamental to the role of any player in an organizational system. It is the obligation of each individual, just as it is the requisite of each team, to focus on growth, development, maturation, and systems advancement in a way that facilitates the achievement of meaningful outcomes and the advancement of patient service. Through the use of systems thinking processes, new mental models, mastering personal skills and relationships within the context of the team, and developing assured focus on outcomes and their advancement are all components of a learning activity. They should be imbedded at every level of learning at the point-of-service in individuals and in teams and reflected in the learning plan in a way that advances the purposes and services of the organization (Box 7-5).

BUILDING AN INFORMATION INFRASTRUCTURE

None of the processes and designs emerging in the health care world could occur at this time if the information systems that make them possible were simply not available. Of the three major initiatives that change the framework for decisions in an organization, perhaps the one with the broadest implications is the information infrastructure.

Technology has made possible radical shifts in relationships, organizations, work, and communication (see Chapter 1). This dramatic growth in the application of technology and work and organizations will continue to have an impact on how work is unfolded, how organizations are defined, and how outcomes are achieved for the foreseeable future. The immediate need for expanding, deepening, and developing the information infrastructure for the continuum of care is important in the design of health care services.

Much of the change in health care reflects an increasing focus on horizontal linkages across a continuum of care with multifocal service providers and a multilateral service population. Within that frame of reference whole new approaches to both organization and structuring design are emerging in the organizational system. Integration of information, as well as integration of service, is a critical part of the effectiveness of organizational design for the future. The information infrastructure is one of the critical elements of that design, requiring much focus on the point-of-service.

Perhaps one of the most intensive difficulties staff members experience as they begin to assume more and more decision making at the point-of-service is the lack of informational support they have in making those decisions. This creates a deficit in the interface of their activities with the activities of the system as a whole.

Clearly, in the old departmental structures the information that was necessary for the department to function could be obtained within the department or by the manager of the department in the course of her or his

BOX **7-5**

Steps to Ownership of Learning

Staff members must own their own development. This is a part of the notion of shifting from looking at work as job toward seeing it more as career. Learning is a lifelong process and does not occur accidentally. Staff members have some obligation for growth:

Step 1: A personal plan of learning is developed with an eye toward career advancement and viability.

Step 2: The fit between personal goals and the system's goals is assessed to determine future response.

Step 3: An action plan that includes a time line is developed to make sure something happens with personal goals.

Step 4: Periodic adjustments occur as circumstances and conditions alter the plan and require changes.

Step 5: Review and evaluate the plan with a trusted colleague or mentor.

Step 6: Get going!

WORDS*of*WISDOM

Information is like a river that flows through the system, carrying with it everything anyone along the river might need to access.

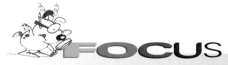

Using the Learning Coach

Staff members should see the learning coach (LC) as a mentor and teacher-learner on the path to creating the learning organization and building effective teams.

- *Use the LC to develop better interactional skills.*
- *Determine personal needs and let the LC help address them.*
- *When communication is a problem, use the LC as a facilitator.*
- *Learn new interpersonal skills and avoid conflict-causing interactions.*
- *As processes fail, use the LC to explore other approaches or options.*
- *The LC role models and mentors different roles and approaches for the staff members, giving them new insights and opportunities.*

Information is not a thing but instead a dynamic. It is a river that flows through an organization and creates the potential for those who need it to reach into the river and draw out whatever is needed in a format that is simple and useful.

relationship with other departmental leaders. The more department structures are deconstructed and service frameworks are moved to the point-of-service, the more integrated the functions and activities of that service become and the greater the demand for information related to those activities emerges at that point-of-service. The challenge in this frame of reference is not only accessed information, but the mix and integration of the information processes necessary to provide specific and definitive support to the team within the context of its expectation and work. Then it must tie the team's work back to the continuum of relationships it has with other service providers and other teams across the continuum of care.

The River of Information

As mentioned previously, information is not a thing, it is a dynamic. Information relates essentially to the processes of access to what is needed to make decisions and to do work.

Information can be characterized in an organizational structure as a "river" flowing through the organization. In that river is contained all the elements necessary to sustain the information base of the organization. The river flows through every component of the system, every service, every team, and every individual and his or her functions throughout the system. It flows in a way in which everything that is possible is present in it. However, it is designed in a way to ensure that only that information that is valued to the individuals who access it at the time they access it is available to them in a way that is useful and viable. A part of the structuring of the river of information through an organization is a clear delineation of just what kind of information is required at what point along the flow or pathway of the river of information as it moves through the organizational system. That way the access to those points at which people dip into the information river and the kind of information that they can use is designed in a way that is specific, clear, and meaningful to the person who draws it out of the river. Although every bit of information is available in the river, access to information must be specifically designed directly to meet the needs of those who access it at the point at which they are located along the pathway of the information river. Therefore managers who are obligated to look at issues related to systems as a whole may gather information from the river on resources, budgets, strategic plans, demographic and geographic indicators, and so forth that are specific and unique to their needs as they look at the system as a whole. The clinical provider, however, at the point-of-service in the system, dipping into the same river, may wish to access entirely different issues. Issues around the continuum of care, critical paths, best practices, the cost per unit of service, the measurement of quality indices, and outcome determinance all are issues of concern to those at the point-of-service. The river contains both those sets of information, but access is designed to help individuals access only that which has meaning for them as they unfold their work and make decisions at their point of decision making in the organizational system. This notion of information as a river creates a dynamic and a process of thinking about information which influences how it will be designed and incorporated into the organizational system. Using this mindset builds requisites around the whole notion of the design of the information infrastructure across the organizational system.

New Tools for Information Management

Focusing on the information infrastructure also assists us in issues around the communication and management of information and data across the system. At the point-of-service, fluidity, flexibility, and mobility are critical factors for the provider. Providers must follow the patient population wherever that patient population is and must be able to quickly access information that facilitates their ability to serve the patient. Therefore affordability becomes critical to the process of making decisions at the point-of-service. Laptop computers, cellular phones, decentralized information stations, patient-based data collection tools, pager tools, documentation, and personal digital assistance are all tools that have meaning and usefulness for those at the point-of-service. These tools provide linkage to the broader river of information, but also provide localized data facilities that ensure the practitioner has adequate resources and maintains her or his mobility in their application (Box 7-6).

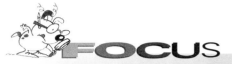

FOCUS

Evidence That You Have a Learning Organization

1. Staff members feel safe to address issues and concerns publicly.
2. Administrators demonstrate their commitment by being learners themselves and are seen in learning roles as learners.
3. Teams are able to deal with their issues free of control or coercion from "above."
4. A lot of time and resources are devoted to development activities.
5. Mistakes are looked at as opportunities for improvement, not as sources of punishment.
6. Learning plans for individuals and teams form the driving force behind growth and improvement in the system.
7. People are rewarded for risk taking, and experimentation is honored by leadership.

BOX 7-6

Providing Information

Teams depend on good information to make decisions. The system must make sure the team can access the information it needs to make good decisions. The system provides for the following:

1. Good information systems leadership who recognize that they are servants to the staff. Their information is only as good as those who can use it.
2. Information must be in a form and a type that can be used at the point-of-service.
3. Information is a constant, not to be managed, but to be generated to as many as will benefit from it.
4. Information is in a language that the user can understand and apply.
5. The hardware is useful and user-friendly, as well as portable.
6. All information must be timely and immediately useful.

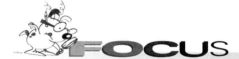

WORDS*of* WISDOM

The individual is obligated to be informed. Communication is a two-way street. Each of us must wants to be informed to the same level as others want to inform us. Both process and desire for communication is necessary for it to happen. You cannot inform someone who does not want to know.

At the management level of the information support system mobility is less important than comprehensiveness. The service manager wants information readily available in a multilateral desktop format that provides service pathway data in a meaningful and viable way that facilitates making judgments immediately about shifts in resources, focus, functions, or activity within the patient pathway. Reporting on demographic and geographic changes, budgetary and financial considerations, revenue changes and adjustments, patient case, acuity, mix, changes, cost and payment base changes, service changes, outcome, and consumer demand shifts and adjustments all provide information that gives a comprehensive composite of data to the manager. This occurs in a way that allows her or him to make reasonable decisions in a relatively abbreviated time frame and that influences both present practice and the future delivery of health care within the service pathway. These examples, one of point-of-service design and the other of service management design, indicate the major shifts in the

FOCUS

For the manager, comprehensive access to a broad database is necessary to his or her work. The ability to "hook into" all of the relevant data sources easily is critical to the effectiveness of the role. Computer-based approaches are necessary. The manager should have at least a desktop computer and access to the financial, service, and strategic data affecting her or his role and service.

- *The manager should be at least computer literate.*
- *All financial data should be coming directly to the service manager.*
- *Data should be both accurate and timely.*
- *Information should be in a form that can be understood by the user.*
- *The manager should know how to use the data effectively.*

need for information and, therefore, the hardware mechanisms and structures of information promulgation in the organizational system.

Increasingly, the dynamics of information generation, data system, and hardware enhancements continually improve the viability of information management systems. An open approach to information management design allows for multiplatform connections, future technology innovations, fluidity in software design, and a flexibility and mobility in the utilization of the technology and the collection and use of data related to it. Building that into the management information infrastructure becomes a critical component ensuring that the information system in place has viability and meaning within the structures of the organization.

As identified in a range of sources, the capital commitment to developing information infrastructure within the health care system over the next decade is considerable. More than 50% of the capital resources of any integrated health care system over the next decade will be in some measure devoted to developing the information infrastructure that supports the continuum of care in a horizontally linked organizational system.

As those resources are being made available, the hardware and tools of information management are becoming increasingly more broad based and less expensive as time moves on. The per unit of cost for information technology is decreasing daily, so the technology is becoming increasingly affordable as it becomes more generalizable across organizational systems. Health care leadership has much to do to begin to apply the emerging technology and the information infrastructure to design of work and of communication within the health care organization. As facility for it becomes more amenable, even the requirement for teams to meet periodically with regard to their activities around critical paths, best practices, clinical outcomes, and evaluation processes will be made much easier. This is facilitated by communication modalities, which allow people to meet in their own offices or clinical settings across an organizational system so that meetings can be undertaken and evaluation sessions can be provided without having to be present in the same location (Box 7-7). Such tele-linkages increasingly facilitate our mobility without eliminating our connectivity.

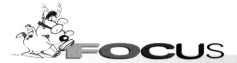

FOCUS

Communication And Information Access

Everyone in the organization has an obligation to access and be aware of the information necessary to do his or her work and to remain current about the conditions and circumstances influencing the organization and its work. The system has an obligation to provide information in a timely and appropriate way. Staff members have a responsibility to stay informed:

Technique 1: *Read memos and bulletins at the beginning of the workday.*

Technique 2: *Have information placed in an individual mailbox for your review.*

Technique 3: *Arrange the bulletin board so that priority, "must read" items stand out so staff will see them clearly.*

Technique 4: *Place important information or notices in the paycheck envelope.*

Technique 5: *Have important information brought up at the beginning or end of the regular staff meeting.*

BOX **7-7**

Technology for Effective Communication

Using technology is important to effective communication. Teams should be able to communicate with each other regardless of where they are located through use of

- E-mail
- Laptop computers
- Modems
- Cellular phones
- Beepers
- Walkie-talkies
- Personal digital assistants
- Internet

Whether local or distant, the technology makes it possible to be in touch with anyone anywhere. Increasing use of these devises on the unit, in the system, or in the community makes communication easier.

CLINICAL INFORMATION AT THE POINT-OF-SERVICE

Increasingly critical is information that relates to the clinical process at the point-of-service. Regardless of the model or approach, all team-based clinical activities will require information that will facilitate the team's decision making in terms of rendering patient care services and adjusting that patient care based on what the data generates regarding outcome and viability of process. Increasingly, immediate information around the process and delivery of the plan of care will be critical to the providers that make up specific teams devoted to define patient populations. Simply because there are teams does not mean that the team members will always be located in the same place at the same time. Their documentation processes must provide a way of linking team members through information with regard to the activities of individual team members, the impact of those activities on the patient, and the intersection those activities have on the activities of any other individual clinical team member.

These circumstances create the condition for a moderated and well-planned patient documentation system that ties into the prevailing information infrastructure. Not only must documentation interface well along the critical clinical continuum of care, it must also integrate with the financial and cost base data that relates to the viability of clinical activities. Obviously, service that cannot be paid for cannot be rendered. Therefore a tightness of fit between the kinds of services that are offered and the payment structure that enumerates them must be clearly delineated. These judgments must be made in short order. Therefore the organization of documentation and data must be such that decisions about the interface of activities and the efficacy of those activities can be made quickly by those who provide leadership along the continuum of care.

It is also important that the interface between the various professionals be facilitated by the information system. Clearly the plan of care for individual consumers, regardless of where they may be located, needs to be facilitated within the context of the expectations and outcomes that are generated. As critical paths and best practices become even better enumerated over the next decade, the plan of care will be more clearly delineated for each of the practitioners within a team-based framework. Therefore the plan of care will indicate for all team members their expectations and activities as they fulfill the obligations of rendering service. In addition, as each provider documents that component that relates to his or her function or validates in the plan of care a component that has been completed, it builds the database for evaluating the efficacy as well as the interface between each of the providers on the team. Increasingly, as the clinical paths and best practice frameworks become more clearly delineated and the role of each practitioner becomes better articulated, the need for a well-defined, clearly integrated information and documentation system will be important to the viability of the practitioner's work and the effectiveness of the team.

The work of the time in building information systems is the linkage between components of the information system. No longer can information leadership look at building information systems without seeing the whole system and its interface and uses. Integrating information is as important as integrating patient care.

The role of information is to create a linkage between people and systems that is fast, fluid, and flexible.

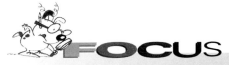

FOCUS

Solving Information Problems

Step 1: *Make sure you know the nature of your problem from the perspective of how it is affecting you now.*

Step 2: *Clearly document the nature of the problem as it occurs so time and circumstances do not alter your vision of the issue.*

Step 3: *Make sure that if anyone else is experiencing a problem, he or she is included in the documentation.*

Step 4: *Go to the source and get the right help in problem solving. If the problem is not the user, either the software or the hardware is the issue.*

Step 5: *After corrective action has occurred, follow up with the source so that he or she can use your experience to help someone else when needed.*

Interfacing Information across the Continuum

As hospitals become health systems and health systems become focused on designing care around subscriber-based continua of services, the importance of the information infrastructure will become critical to the sustainability of such systems. As health care becomes more subscriber driven and the continuum becomes the basic framework for health care delivery, integration along that continuum in a horizontally linked structure will become the modus operandi for functioning in the system. This will often mean that organizations will be linked and connected to other providers of patient services that they neither own nor control. Creating linkage across the continuum of care within a system is indeed challenging. What is especially difficult is creating those same linkages across the continuum of care, interfacing with those parts of the continuum that are not a subset of the system; however, such linkages will be necessary.

Partners must be able to share specific and appropriate clinical information regarding patient populations they are expected to serve. They have the same right to a broad-based database that influences the judgments and activities of their providers at that particular point in the continuum. Therefore designing systems that make it flexible and fluid enough for partners becomes an important part of the consideration around building an effective information infrastructure. The linkage of the documentation system, the design of the continuum of services, and the generation of patient-based information all become important parts of the dynamic of building an effective organizational and informational interface.

However, distinguishing the kind of information means also designing it in a way that has value and is viable for the provider at a specific time or point along the continuum of care. For example, the kinds of information that are required of home health professionals are not the same information as required of rehabilitation professionals. Further, the information generated within the women's services pathway of a health care system might not be nearly as valuable when an individual patient moves across the continuum into cancer care services. Yet all of these services need to be easily accessible to those components of the documentation process that are critical to their clinical activities within a context that gives them a complete enough picture of the patient and the patient's circumstances in a way that facilitates service delivery (Box 7-8).

Each of these issues regarding information from management, the clinical system, teams, individual clinical providers, and across the continuum of care has tremendous implications for design, character, and quality of the information infrastructure. Clearly, the information infrastructure is the architecture for the future of health care. Therefore consideration of its design must be a major construct of the work of the team-based organization. The only way in which team-based decision-making and point-of-service orientation can be maintained over the long term is through the kind and quality of the development of the information infrastructure that supports it. This river of information creates the continuing viability on which systems, organizational, operational, and clinical viability can be advanced (Box 7-9).

BOX **7-8**

Documentation Notes
• As much as possible, documentation should occur in the electronic record.   • The clinical path should be the foundation for the clinical record.   • Interdisciplinary processes are the foundation for all patient activities.   • The design of the electronic record should make documentation easier and faster.   • Information should be concise yet comprehensive.   • The patient's service pathway is the foundation for information generation.   • Hardware should be easy to use.   • All hardware should be portable and flexible to use.   • Clinical and financial information should be available at the same time in the same documents.   • Providers should be able to chart easily and have access to each other's information quickly.

BOX **7-9**

Critical Information That Supports the Team's Work
1. The team is the basic unit of interdisciplinary communication.   2. All information about the patient is generated to facilitate the work of patient care.   3. Financial data is always support to the clinical data, not the reverse.   4. Information helps the provider guide the patient across the continuum of services.   5. All information about the patient is available to the patient at all times.   6. Information provides the data necessary to create a tightness-of-fit between patient and provider.   7. Information helps the team evaluate the effectiveness of patient service strategies.

Building Relationships between Teams

This book focuses on effective team functioning. The characteristic of that effectiveness is the relationship that exists between and among teams. For the most part teams develop within the contexts of their own pathways. The number, kind, and character of teams is determined by the complexity, breadth, and character of the pathway itself. In pathways where there is a relatively narrow frame of reference with regard to services, there are few team differences along the pathway. However, in those pathways where there is a tremendous amount of variability and clinical work, such as in women's health or behavioral services, there are widely variable teams, depending on the patient's needs, the locus of service, and the breadth of services that are offered by the system. Also influencing effectiveness is the communication of teams across pathways as subscribers or patients move from one clinical pathway to another, driven by circumstances or clinical condition. Here again, the information infrastructure is critical to cross-pathway team communication. Although the interface of the teams is relatively limited and short term, the communication of essential information, clinical activities, and issues regarding patient needs is a predominant focus of communication across pathways. This can be supported through the effective design of the clinical information system and the method for documenting care.

Team-based relationships will become vitally important within pathways. Moving the patient along a continuum of care within a clinical pathway demands that teams are able to communicate effectively within a pathway along that continuum of care. The information infrastructure is certainly of value to ensure that the documentation of services along the continuum is clearly enumerated, well identified, and communicated effectively. Still, mechanisms for relationships and building a strong service interface along the continuum are important to the effectiveness of the clinical pathway.

A focus on the following issues is important to the effectiveness of team-based relationship along the continuum within specific service pathways.

Teams cannot function independently of each other. In a continuum of services the interaction between teams is critical to the patient flow through the service system. Every team has a need to interact with others along the continuum of care and requires as much support in the process from each other as needed to facilitate the patient's flow through the system.

No one falls outside a relationship with teams in the system. The team connects the system to the patient. It is through the team that problems are identified and solved. All supports are designed to facilitate the effectiveness of the team. Anything in the system that does not support the team will always impede it.

1. The service pathway has a clear mechanism for interfacing team leadership from the pathway across the continuum in making policy decisions regarding patient flow and communication strategies.
2. A continuum-based communication design, constructed by the pathway council (made up of team leadership and other team members), whose purpose is to ensure effective communication flow across the pathway and identification of problems and issues associated with implementing, exists.
3. The pathway has in place a mechanism for continually assessing the quality of communication and the flow of patients along the continuum of care between teams and within the pathway as a whole. Design of an effective evaluation system keeps team leadership focused on identifying and resolving issues that constrain team interface as a part of the team's ongoing and operational obligations.
4. Resolving problems in patient flow that relate not only to team interface within the pathway but intersection with diagnostic and therapeutic services that fall outside of the pathway is a critical part of flow problem resolution. Leadership from diagnostic and therapeutic services not aligned to the pathway is involved at the point-of-service with team leaders to resolve issues of flow and interface with services around the patient pathway. The frequency of these sessions is driven by data that generates out of the evaluation process.
5. Team members must have the opportunity to evaluate the efficacy of the information system in relationship to three issues: (1) access; (2) the viability of the data; and (3) how it facilitates the mobility and interaction of the providers. The information infrastructure will go far in eliminating many of the database problems affecting patient flow. However, unresolved issues related to information generation can create critical noise along the patient's pathway and between and among team members.

Finally, it is important that problems or issues of concern between and among teams that relate to relationships, personalities, competence, or ef-

All decisions regarding the work of the team should be made by the team. All issues with regard to clinical activities and standards belong to the team. Performance expectations regarding the work should be clear and consistent for all team members.

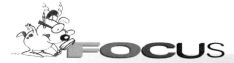

The key purposes of clinical teams are to:
1. Integrate the providers around specific patient populations
2. Configure providers to create a horizontal linkage to each other to make communication easier and better
3. Link the work of essential providers around one standard of service and plan of care
4. Focus the energy and work of providers on their service, not on trying to survive the system
5. Bring decision makers together to create efficiencies and improve the "fit" of their decisions with each other
6. Strengthen the work relationships between providers, focusing them on the mutual outcomes and supportive processes

Teams have a horizontal perspective, seeing their relationship across the system rather than up and down the system. Relationship (horizontal) in teams is more important than control (vertical).

The team is the focal point of accountability. Team members are obligated to develop their skills in decision making and in unfolding their work. The ability to achieve sustainable outcomes depends on the team's willingness to own its work and the outcomes it produces.

fectiveness also be addressed as a part of the service pathways operation. Performance evaluation should also look not only at the team function, but at the interface of team activity within the pathway itself. Focusing at the performance of the pathway helps orient the minds of clinical leaders in the pathway council regarding the efficiency and effectiveness of the pathway. This occurs in light of the outcomes the team achieves in facilitating the patient's journey, enhancing the experience of the patient along the continuum, and meeting the clinical outcomes anticipated through the patient's experience with the clinical pathway. This gives a frame of reference to the teams that is broader than the work of any one team and orients the mindsets of team leaders around their relationship within the context of the patient's pathway. In this way the team focuses less on its identity with regard to its own membership and more on its identity and relationship with the pathway and the patients it is directed to serve.

THE CLINICAL MODEL OF SERVICE DELIVERY

Any organization that wishes to create a sustainable framework for delivering its service must operate within the context of models that result in excellent practice, with normative outcomes of high level of satisfaction and ideal levels of health for its subscribers. Building team-based approaches to care should affect clinical performance, resource use, the quality of outcomes, the character of service, and the speed with which subscribers can obtain what they need from the system. Within this frame of reference the design of the care model or critical activities of care becomes critical to the organizational system.

Processes associated with reengineering and restructuring the system become the framework within which new approaches to delivering care unfold. Clearly there must be a model within which the system unfolds its care and evaluates the effectiveness of that care as it begins to define the character of its system. Within the context of that framework that model must interface well with the priorities and strategies of the system. The model must build around the consumers to whom it has directed its service structure, and it must build an organizational structure that supports the kind and character of service it provides to its community of users. Several components to the delivery of care must be identified to ensure that care delivery can unfold.

The three basic components of the care delivery model are the care delivery framework, interdisciplinary relationships, and the growth of practice in the system. These are the cornerstones on which the care delivery system can be renewed and continually addressed within the context of meaningful and viable patient care outcomes.

Elements of the Model of Care Delivery

A number of issues must be addressed regarding care delivery to make sure that all components of care are undertaken and incorporated within the context of team-based behaviors. Each team will have an obligation for developing its functions and activities and for clarifying its critical paths and continua of services, its responsibilities, and its quality requirements, as well as its clear delineation of the accountabilities of various players within the care delivery system (Box 7-10). Each of these elements is important to

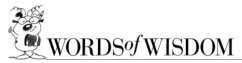

WORDS *of* WISDOM

Giving teams obligations without accountability and authority ensures that the team will not succeed. Most of the decisions made in the new health systems have to be driven from the point-of-service. The members of the team must have both the skills and the ability to make effective decisions affecting the functioning of the system. They must have the power necessary to make them!

⁓

BOX 7-10

Managers will have to help teams interface well with each other by:
1. Identifying barriers to their communication across the system
2. Breaking down control systems that keep teams from accessing each other easily
3. Facilitating the construction and generation of good information, which helps the teams work better and more efficiently
4. Identifying conflict early and working to short-circuit it before it becomes a serious impediment
5. Removing departmental "silos" that limit access and communication across the system
6. Making sure that teams have the right information to make good decisions
7. Evaluating the effectiveness of the team's relationships both inside and outside the team

Designing the model of care at the point-of-service is the most critical activity of any team. The approach to providing service is one of the most transparent ways for patients to evaluate the quality of the care from their perspective.

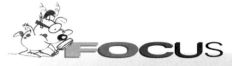

FOCUS

Do You Have Trouble Connecting Teams?

If you have trouble connecting teams, perhaps one of the following is at work:

- *No real communication method has been incorporated into your team's function.*
- *The teams see no reason yet to be connected to each other.*
- *The managers are not getting along.*
- *Team members are not working well together.*
- *The continuum of care between the teams is still not well defined.*
- *Teams do not like each other.*
- *There has been no expectation that the teams communicate. The skills necessary to interrelate are not yet present.*
- *The teams are in their formative stages and still need some time to develop.*

the design of the system in a way that addresses the effectiveness of both those who provide the service and the system itself as it provides the framework for that system.

Perhaps the cornerstones of the elements of care processing are those critical paths or care delivery components that 90% of the time can be clearly articulated around which each member of the team can configure his or her practice. If point-of-service delivery is to achieve advancement of clinical practice and to move decision making to that point-of-service in pursuance of that goal, obviously mechanisms must be in place that address changes in current practice to create integrative models of practice.

Developing Tools

A framework or format must have incorporated into it standards of service or care, accountability delineation of each of the providers on the team, the quality of measures that indicate performance against the expectations, and the aggregated responsibility of the team. The team must commit to achieving the outcomes it determines best represents what can be done within the context of delivering service. This approach to delivering care organizes and systematizes it in a way in which the critical paths or best practice framework can result from the delivery of service in a meaningful way that can be continued and replicated over a number of patients within the same pathway.

Clearly, the goal of defining a system for care delivery is to ensure that the desired outcomes are achieved and replicated in patients over the pathway continuously. Therefore the following questions arise in the design of care delivery:

- What practices or activities can best reproduce the outcomes expected?
- What is the clinical decision process that supports that?
- Who makes those decisions?
- What are their relationships to each other?
- How clear are their activities in relationship to each other?

- How are they documented in the information infrastructure to make sure that the activities, functions, and processes associated with care result in some measurable and meaningful outcome that can be visualized and evaluated by all members of the team?

The patient is the center of all activities in defining response to patient need. Focusing on the patient's pathway for the continua of services required within the pathway means understanding the patient's needs all across the setting, and what activities will be necessary to meet those needs within the cost as well as the service framework available. To avoid fragmentation of service integration of the activities of the professionals must be identified in the care system.

Increasingly, issues of case management—managing the patient's continuum, mapping the services that are necessary to ensure the patient's

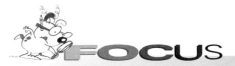

Team Development Stages

Stage 1: Team role and purpose are worked out with the members.

Stage 2: Team relationships, rules, and interactions are defined early in team formation.

Stage 3: The work elements, critical paths, protocols, and outcome delineations are defined and refined for implementation and evaluation.

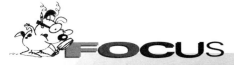

Leadership needs to ensure that the team can enumerate its accountabilities for patient care and will follow through with expectations.

Stage 1: There is a clearly defined set of team expectations for each member's role.

Stage 2: Team is clear about its accountability for patient care and the authority it has to make decisions.

Stage 3: There are good monitors for assessing the congruence of the team with its role and results.

Stage 4: Corrective action strategies are clear and timely when response is required.

Stage 5: The standard of excellence identified and achieved by the team can be replicated, and the team is able to raise the standard.

needs are met, and evaluating the relationship between process and outcome to determine tightness of fit—are significant parts of clarifying the care delivery components necessary to an effective team-based system.

At the pathway level team membership must focus on a clinical system that represents the accountability of each of the teams along the continuum of care so that each team is addressing its component of service along the patient's pathway. Therefore the pathway leadership needs to focus on the following issues:

1. How is patient care coordinated across the continuum for a similar group of patients who require a specific series of activities to meet their needs?
2. How does leadership make sure that each of the teams continually achieves consistent processes across the continuum of care that result in a tight fit between the processes and the outcomes?
3. How does each team ensure that the mix and outlay of resources is appropriate to the demand of service within the context of the critical path it has constructed for specific patient populations?
4. What mechanisms are put in place at the team level to ensure an ongoing evaluation of the effectiveness of the team's work and an ability to intervene immediately when the processes or the outcomes do not evidence a high level of fit?
5. Evaluate the effectiveness of each team member's role and function within the context of the team expectation for that member's functions, activities, and performance. Each of these provides the framework for ensuring that the activities of all team members fit the prevailing design and expectation for service within each critical path or best practice determined within the pathway.

Clearly, the move to best practice indicates the pathway's commitment to use of a systems approach to delivering patient care. Through the development of the best practice format a consistent framework is provided within which the performance of both team and individual members can be clearly enumerated. Incorporating this into the information infrastructure and creating a documentation system that supports the best practice

Teams represent the organization's commitment to the belief that it comprises a community of knowledge workers who have converged around a common purpose to achieve excellent clinical outcomes.

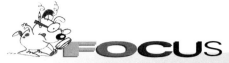

Keeping the patient at the center of the team's work is a necessity if a sustainable outcome is to be achieved. Some organizations have unique ways of ensuring that happens:

- *The patient is directly involved in specific care planning with the providers.*
- *Patients are a part of designing the critical paths for each clinical service.*
- *Patients are asked to evaluate their experience within the care path format.*
- *Patients are a part of the team evaluation of its own role and behavior toward patients.*
- *Patient's family members assess the team's responsiveness to them and their incorporation into care activities.*

format and can be used for evaluating the effectiveness of the team's approach to care delivery strengthens the ability to deliver the service, replicate the standards, and evaluate the effectiveness of care delivery. To ensure that a thorough and consistent approach around care delivery has been defined, incorporated in each of the components must be issues that relate to the use of resources, the accountability of each of the providers within the context of the team, the outcomes expected of each team, the standards that are consistently applied both from the disciplines and when aggregated by the team as a whole, and the measurement and evaluation of outcomes within the framework of specific patient populations.

Interdisciplinary Practice

Effectiveness within a clinical model cannot be obtained without mechanisms in place that address the requisites of interdisciplinary relationship.

TEAM**TIP**   7.2

Partnership

The best way to teach partnership to others (including doctors) is to model it in your own behavior. If true and sustainable partnership between team members is evident, others will soon recognize it and seek to relate to you. In the face of stressors, real partners pull together instead of fall apart. Unity is the sign of vigor in real partnerships.

Issues around communication, documentation, normative practice standards, shared decision making, and team-based relations are all elements that must be incorporated into the interdisciplinary framework for practice. Models should relate to building the relationship between the disciplines at the team level and across the pathway. They should interface with the learning plan and the individual agendas at the team level. Models should also work at the pathway level for building a learning dynamic that results in stronger relationships and a clearer configuration of the teams and individuals around best practices and clearly delineated patient outcomes.

Perhaps the most difficult component of integration of the disciplines will be around integrating physicians into the disciplinary framework. A number of changes occurring in health care will facilitate the integration of physicians across the continuum of care (Team Tip 7-2). These elements of change are creating some of the preconditions that will help pathway and team leadership in the process of coordinating and integrating physician practices into the team-based process.

Physicians do not learn partnered practices as a part of their developmental process (see Chapter 1). Therefore part of a learning plan will be devoted to developing skills of physicians in partnership arrangements out of unilateral individualistic entrepreneurial approaches to health care practice. Increasingly, payment structures, service frameworks, and organizational designs are built on the assumption that the physician will be a more integral part of the team-based approach to delivering care. The partnership of the physician is critical to the sustenance and advancement of care delivery in a subscriber-based organizational system. The role of pathway leadership, as well as team members, is to facilitate as much as possible the journey of the physician from individualistic nonaligned practice frameworks to partnership team-based approaches to care delivery. This requires participation and education, mentoring and networking, partnering activities, facilitating the transition in behavioral patterns, and persevering in a relatively emotionally charged and challenging process of building relationships that have not previously been configured in a team-based framework.

Although it is clearly the obligation of all professional services and disciplines to be building the relationship, physicians are the most difficult because of the traditional relationship the physician has had with the health care system. However, elements of difficulty with regard to physicians are imbedded in developing relationships between and among all practitioners. The challenges in building structures, learning processes, support systems, accountability expectations, and demands on individuals and teams is ensuring that collaborative and integrative practices become the model of care delivery and service relationship at the point-of-service and across the continuum of care within any given health system.

To build the high-performance, team-based relationships that are necessary, focus on the following elements will be critical to developing effectiveness:

1. Individuals must know that their own development and learning is a lifelong process that is a continual expectation of their growing, practice, activities, and relationships.

2. Individuals must recognize that there must be a match between their knowledge base and skill enhancement and the strategic and learning goals of the organizational system to ensure that there is a fit between the individual performance of the practitioner and the outcome expectations of the team.

3. Individuals have an increasing obligation for dialogue, negotiation, conflict resolution, problem solving, and solution seeking. This must unfold in each one's relationship to the other as a part of the team-based group dynamics.

4. Every individual member of the team is expected to focus on outcomes. The relationship between the team member's activities and outcomes to which they are directed must always give form to the thinking and functioning of every team member.

5. No practices are constant or continuous or exempt of the requisites of change. Outcomes will define the viability of any individual or team action. Adjustment of activities and functions both at the team and the in-

TEAM DEVELOPMENTAL CYCLE

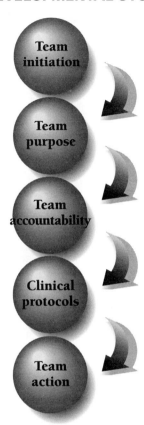

Team members must be able to function across their disciplinary boundaries. Each discipline believes it is guiding the others across the continuum of service. The truth is, no one has responsibility for someone else. Each team member has a specific role and contribution to make, which must be clear and for which each member must be accountable.

The goal of the team is to ensure that the best practice of the providers is available to those it serves. Real value demands that the best balance between resources required and care needed be achieved by those who do the work of care. Team members must live that relationship in all they do.

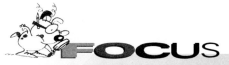

FOCUS

Physicians are no longer outside the cycle of accountability and relationship. The team is now the format for all clinical relationships. It will take time and effort to help physicians operate as members of the team rather than "captains" of the process:

- Bring willing doctors into the teams first.
- Build doctor involvement around clinical process, not administrative activity.
- Put the patient at the center of the team's focus and dialogue.
- Use the "best practice" approach to keep doctors interested.
- Make sure the physician has clear accountability and that the team has some expectations for performance.
- Hold the doctor to his or her accountability, and reinforce the doctor's membership on the team.

dividual level will be required as the outcome delineations demand such adjustments.

Each of the above addresses both team and individual performance. Here again, the tightness of fit between the individual and the team activity and the activities of the team with the pathway are critical moderators of the successful unfolding of a team-based approach to delivery of care within the model of care. The team's commitment and the individual's activities must resonate with each other around the care delivery process, the best practice framework that has been developed within the service pathway. This tightness of fit is the measure of the effectiveness, efficiency, and viability of the team-based approach to care delivery.

CONTINUING DEVELOPMENT AND THE ADVANCEMENT OF PRACTICE

Commitment to individual and team learning are essential to the viability of team-based approaches and point-of-service design. However, it is not only the individual commitment to this process that needs to be stressed. The system's commitment to the advancement of practice within the model of care delivery is important to the integrity of patient care services (Box 7-11). At the service pathway level within the context of the team and with individuals' continuing commitment to the advancement of practice, the development of knowledge and the consonance of individual behaviors with the learning plan are critical elements in the successful unfolding of a model for care delivery.

As best practices continue to unfold and get better defined in the information system, they serve as the database for advancing the knowledge, practice, and understanding of individual team members and of the team as a whole around the needs for continual learning. Indeed they identify the content of continual learning that will need to be the focus of learning activities of each member of the team, as well as the team as a whole. Standards of practice cannot be advanced or raised without a concomitant improvement in the practice activities and standards of those who unfold practice. Therefore continuing attention to the learning equation and to developing the activities of clinical practice around the continuum of care becomes important work at the team level and at the pathway level within each service pathway.

The scope of learning and the activities related to learning depend entirely on the issues that center around the following questions:

1. How tight is the fit between what I know as a practitioner and the demand being placed on my role?
2. What do the outcomes of our best practice approach to delivering care and the care model tell me about my contribution to them?
3. What plan of growth do I have for my own career to position me to be more viable in the delivery of health care services and as a team member?
4. What deficits in the outcome of care form the foundation for a learning plan that affects my own practice and my own learning strategies?
5. What is the learning plan for the service pathway, and how does my individual learning plan fit the demands of team development, the improvement of the care delivery model, and my own performance as a member of the clinical care team?
6. What is my long-term goal for learning, development, and career advancement?

The above questions form the framework for an individual team member's obligation for addressing her or his own learning within the context of the service pathway and the team's function. Also, these questions tie the activities of the individual to the clinical model. The model of care delivery, the best practices that enumerate it, the relationships between and among the providers, the fit of clinical process with the desired outcomes of care, levels of patient satisfaction, and the evidence that suggests the high quality practice at the team level all serve as the template within which the individuals practice. This has an impact on the team's activities and relationships and the service pathway's commitment to the continuum of care.

BOX 7-11

Advancing Practice

It is the responsibility of every professional to advance the practice of his or her profession. The services that are provided to patients will be enhanced and improved by
- Raising standards of practice
- Improving patient services
- Enhancing the quality of care
- Challenging rituals and routines
- Advancing expectations for performance
- Producing higher-level outcomes

The real value of the work of the team is always evidenced in the outcomes it achieves, not the processes it puts in place. As with everything in life the results of work give evidence of its value.

The objective of the system is to bring into a high degree of congruence the intent of the individual professional and the purposes of the organization. Each is committed to service; therefore both must have the same goals for those they serve.

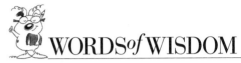

WORDS of WISDOM

Building the future occurs with each little act that responds to each day's changes.

INTEGRATED SERVICE SYSTEM

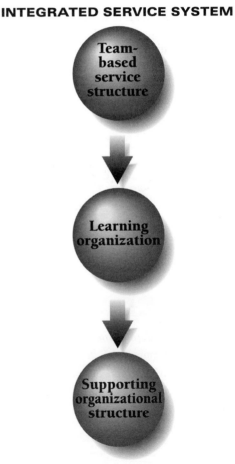

Team-based service structure

Learning organization

Supporting organizational structure

Each component of a service delivery system has a direct and abiding relationship to each other and an impact on each other. Indeed, they provide a seamless linkage across the continuum of service that affects the way decisions are made and the sustenance of the organization around the subscriber for whom the service is designed and the system is configured.

Each of these arenas of decision making affects the efficacy and viability of the service provided by the organization. It is the obligation of leadership not only to see the relationship between them, but to build the constructs which ensure that they operate in a continuous and effective way. The system's ultimate obligation is to support its mission and purposes. Further, all elements of the system must converge to render support for that mission and purpose.

Ultimately, the purpose of any service system is to provide service to the subscribers who use it to create a tightness of fit between the structures of service and those who receive it. This seamless interface between each of the components outlined in this chapter is a foundational requisite for the effectiveness of an integrated point-of-service and team-based delivery system. In conjunction with the other elements of team-based approaches identified in this book it forms the foundation for system success.

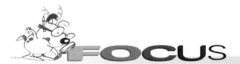

FOCUS

The model of care should reflect all the processes and structures that led to it. Included in the model are all the elements of:
- *Standards of practice*
- *Dialogue between the disciplines*
- *Protocols*
- *Specific role expectations*
- *Team-driven processes*
- *Critical path work*
- *Outcome delineations*

Bibliography

Baker J: They may want to take charge, but can physicians really organize? *Journal of Health Care Finance* 21(3):6-8, 1995.

Barting A: Integrated delivery systems: fact or fiction, *Healthcare Executive* 10(3):6-11, 1995.

Cave D: Vertical integration models to prepare health systems for capitation, *Health Care Management Review* 20(1): 26-39, 1995.

Coeling H, Wilcox J: Steps to collaboration, *Nursing Administration Quarterly* 18(4): 44-55, 1994.

Coile R: *Five stages of managed care,* Chicago, Health Administration Press, 1997.

D'Aprix R: *Communicating for change,* San Francisco, Jossey-Bass, 1996.

Doerge J, Hagenow N: Integrating care delivery, *Nursing Administration Quarterly* 20(2): 42-48, 1996.

Griffith J: The infrastructure of integrated delivery systems, *Healthcare Executive* 10(3): 12-17, 1995.

Heskett J et al: Putting the service-profit chain to work, *Harvard Business Review* 72(2): 164-173, 1994.

Hurley R et al: Toward a seamless health care delivery system, *Frontiers of Health Service Management* 9(4):5-44, 1993.

Kaluzny A, Zuckerman H, Ricketts T: Partners for the dance: forming strategic alliances in health care, Chicago, *Health Administration Press,* 1995.

Kim D: *Toward learning organizations,* Cambridge, Mass, Pegasus Communication, 1992.

Larson E: New rules for the game interdisciplinary education for professionals, *Nursing Outlook* 43(4): 180-185, 1995.

Macy J: Collective self interest—the holonic shift, *World Business Academy Perspectives* 9(1): 19-22, 1995.

Maynard H, Mehrtens S: *The fourth wave: business in the 21st century,* San Francisco, Berrett-Koehler, 1993.

Meighan S: Managing conflict in an integrated system, *Topics in Health Care Financing* 20(4): 39-47, 1994.

Moore N, Komras H: *Patient focused healing,* San Francisco, Jossey-Bass, 1993.

Parker G: *Team players and teamwork,* San Francisco, Jossey-Bass, 1993.

Patterson Hines P, Smeltzer C, Galletti M: Work restructuring: the process of redefining the role of patient caregiver, *Nursing Economics* 12(6): 346-350, 1994.

Porter-O'Grady T: Whole systems shared governance: creating the seamless organization, *Nursing Economics* 12(4): 187-195, 1994.

Tan J: Integrating health care with information technology, *Health Care Management Review* 19(2): 72-80, 1994.

TOOLCHEST

TOOL A: Team Meeting Checklist

All meetings should have a framework and a format for their unfolding. All too often health care meetings are called simply to have conversations or to discuss a number of issues with very few guidelines, rules, or processes in place to discipline the meeting framework. Meetings are the keystone for successful group process; therefore setting up for meetings to make them effective and productive is critical. This checklist serves as the foundation for ensuring that all of the elements are in place for effective team meetings.

Instructions for an Effective Team Meeting

Setting Agendas

Every meeting should have a specific agenda. There should not be more than three to five items on the agenda. Any more items than that generally ensures that the meeting cannot be successful in achieving all of its outcomes.

The meeting facilitator should check off the following items in relationship to the agenda:
1. Agenda topics are clear and specific.
2. Those presenting at the meeting have been clearly identified and know what they are doing.
3. A timeline has been established for each agenda item.

4. Each item has been identified as either requiring discussion, making decision, or simply for information.

Facilitator's Role

Every meeting should have an informed, capable facilitator able to guide the meeting through its activities. The facilitator should be able to check off the following:
1. The agenda is concise, brief, and appropriate.
2. The timeline has been clearly identified and will be adhered to.
3. The ability to get dialogue and discussion from each participant is acknowledged. Disciplined dialogue processes are incorporated into the process of the meeting.

Minutes

Minutes should be provided. They should be as brief and as complete as possible. The best format for minutes is bullet model rather than paragraphic design. The minutes should represent the following items:
1. Describe in the minutes each of the agenda items identified with action included.

2. Specific points or items related to the agenda should be enumerated in the meeting.
3. Individuals making key points or moving for decisions should be identified.
4. A continuous format for minutes should be adopted early in the meeting process.
5. As much as possible, meeting minute taking should be rotated among members.

Discussion Elements Identified

All discussion should be disciplined and effective. There should be few conversations, long-winded presentations, or diversions from the agenda items in the issues. The following should be used as skills in ensuring effective meeting process:

1. Seeking clarification. All issues should be clarified so that common understanding is achieved from all of the members.
2. Monitoring dialogue. The facilitator should be clear that all participants can be heard from, but that their comments are specific, concise, and to the point of the agenda.
3. Opportunity to listen should be provided in the format of the discussion so that people can hear the exploration of notions or ideas related to the agenda item and respond to them.
4. Summarization. The chair or facilitator should clearly summarize points as they are made before making decisions so that the team understands the content of their discussion.
5. Prevent diversion and digression. The facilitator should ensure that the discussion stays specifically focused on the agenda and related issues. Broad-ranging discussion or conversation should be avoided.
6. Keep to the time frame. Each agenda item has a specific time frame. The facilitator should monitor that time frame, discussion, and related decisions.
7. Find generalized consensus. At the end of a discussion, determination of where the group is in relationship to the issue or decision being made, levels of agreement, and outstanding issues should be identified.
8. Ending the meeting. Following decision, time commitment, or the termination of the meeting, understanding of the activities accomplished at the meeting, where the participants are, and the next meeting time or follow-up of the meeting should be identified by the facilitator consistent with the expectations for the closure of the meeting.
9. Meeting evaluation. The facilitator and key members of the team, observers, or other leaders should momentarily assess the mechanics, dynamics, and process of the meeting to determine its effectiveness and to identify ways in which the next meeting process can be improved.

TOOL B: Team Conflict Resolution Exercise

The purpose of this exercise is to help a team identify and resolve conflict within and among its members to move to solution and to maintaining focus on the work of the team.

- Group size: a team of no more than ten (10) members
- Time: 2 to 3 hours
- Environment: a meeting room with one large table

- Supplies: a flip chart, blackboard, colored pens or markers, and masking tape

Instructions and Activity

The facilitator explains the purpose of the process, identifying as specifically as possible the appearance of the conflict as he or she identifies it. The facilitator outlines various conflict resolution strategies and the impact of unresolved conflict on the dynamics and work of the group.

At the end of the presentation, the group facilitator divides the team into two halves, breaks the team up, and sends them to opposite sides of the room. The team facilitator then asks two questions:

1. What is it about the behavior of the members of the other group that concerns us, creates difficulties with us, or simply impedes with the work of the team? *Note:* Be as specific as possible with regard to the behaviors, but do not identify the individuals.

After deliberating and laying out on the flip chart the answer to the first question, the group asks itself a second question:

2. What is it about us or what we do that creates problems or barriers to group process, consensus building, or problem solving in the group's activity or work? Identify the responses to these in the same way that you identify the responses

to the previous question.

The two group halves come back together again with their flip charts and information. Each group shares the answer to their first question with the other and then follows with the answer to the second question with the other. The group facilitator guides the group through a discussion of the issues and helps them identify the key issues that are the focus of their conflict. The priority conflict issues are identified in this process.

The group breaks up one more time and again takes the priorities identified and begins to strategize the solutions and responses to them and places them on the flip chart. After about 20 minutes of discussion the group returns to the table and brings the results of their discussion with them. The facilitator works with the group to identify the responses to the priorities and to begin to get consensus around actions and activities related to those responses.

The activities are identified, the commitment to undertake them is enumerated, focus on behavioral or group change is identified, a time frame for responding and measuring response is indicated, and the meeting is called to a close. In subsequent meetings the decisions made by this process are identified for evaluation and assessment of progress or adjustment and change.

TOOL C: Team Time Management Profile

Time management is always one of the more critical issues in team process. Team members and teams as a whole generally indicate that time is something that not a lot of people have in surplus. Therefore good time management strategies are

critical to the success of the group. Being able to address the issue of time is also addressing the issue of effectiveness. Therefore this time inventory provides an opportunity for the leadership to focus on the major issues of time and to rate them.

Instructions: In the rating score between 1 and 4 (1—never; 2—sometimes; 3—often; 4—always) the leader should indicate the level of priority of frequency she or he attaches to the time-based activities identified in the profile. The score that she or he gets indicates the kinds of response or priorities she or he should apply to individual time management for managing the team's time.

1. I always set aside appropriate time for the team meeting.
2. I have a tightly planned team agenda to make sure that the team focuses on its work.
3. I know where all of the team papers and documents are and can find them immediately.
4. My schedule incorporates the time spent on team interaction and meeting.
5. I have a clearly defined "to do" list in relationship to team activities.
6. I am able to take on several tasks at one time.
7. I find myself losing sight of short-term goals in the interest of long-term goals.
8. I find myself losing sight of long-term goals in the interest of short-term goals.
9. I am able to stay concentrated at team meetings.
10. I spend time focusing on preparing for the team meeting, to spend less time at the team meeting.
11. I map out the steps of discussion and dialogue in advance of having it, to make good use of time.
12. I establish time frames for each specific agenda item before meetings.
13. I identify four team members' time permitted for discussion.

14. The team identifies specific time goals for each team action.
15. Each team project and activity has a specified time frame.
16. I evaluate critically each team goal and action within the time frame for completing it.
17. I follow up with team members assigned to specific activities to ensure that they are on time.
18. I make sure all team members are present at team processes to ensure general achievement of outcomes in a timely way.
19. I start meetings on time and end them on time.
20. Discussions are specific, to the point, and brief.
21. I always use a flip chart for externalizing the dialogue and identifying key points.
22. Priorities are established efficiently and consistently in the decision-making process.
23. I plan for meeting presentations to be efficient, timely, and to the point.
24. I meet with all personnel presenting at meetings ahead of time to reinforce the timeliness and succinctness of each presentation.
25. I evaluate the effectiveness of each meeting to determine the appropriate use of time.

Each participant should look at the numbers attached to each of the time priorities identified above. If there are a number of 1 and 2 items, prioritizing those in terms of developmental work on the part of the leader will help further refine and develop her or his skills. Using this profile helps focus on developing the skill base for time management in the context of the team format.

TOOLD:Getting the Team Unstuck

J. R. Katzenbach and D. K. Smith* identify that teams can get stuck in their process and need some specific work to be able to move on and continue their work. Several activities on the part of team leaders are required to ensure that the team is able to do its work and to do it without getting stuck on some of the processes that create issues of concern. Following are the most difficult issues that create a sense of being stuck in teams requiring assessment:

1. *A loss of purpose or meaning*
   - Does the team remember why they have gathered together?
   - Is the team clear about what its fundamental work is?
   - Can the team tie its functional activities to its purpose?
   - Has the team been caught in its incremental activities, forgetting the general direction of the team?
   - Are the team's goals still clear?
   - Does the team still understand and agree on why they are working together?
2. *A loss of integrity and commitment*
   - Has conflict caused the team to lose its way?
   - Have team members been diverted by situations and issues between and among members?
   - Have unresolved past issues accumulated so that purpose and meaning have been sidetracked?

- Has the team moved from disciplined dialogue into broad-ranging conversations producing no outcome?
- Have personality, role, and function issues impeded the team's ability to focus?
- Has anger, discord, or conflict become the focus of the team's activities rather than its original purpose and mission?

3. *A diminished skill base*
   - Is the team able to undertake its work?
   - Are team members expressing deficits in their skills to do the work of the team?
   - Is the developmental level of the team sufficient to the activities and work before it?
   - Is the competence of members around team process clear and appropriate?
   - Are the disciplines of dialogue imbedded in the discussions and decisions made by the team?
   - Are the processes and the work of the team consistent with the outcomes expected from the team?
   - Is the team competent to fulfill its purpose?
4. *Inadequate leadership*
   - Are the team's leaders competent to undertake the process of the team?
   - Is the team leadership consistent with the expectations for team process?
   - Are the disciplines of good leadership apparent in the team's leaders?
   - Is the leader competent to undertake the dynamic processes of team dialogue and decision making?
   - Are the personal skills and attributes of the team leader impeding or facilitating team process?

* Katzenbach JR, Smith DK: *The wisdom of teams*, New York, Harper Collins, 1993.

- Are the knowledge level and learning foundations for team leadership apparent in the roles and skills of the leader in the process of teamwork?
- Does the team respect the contributions and role of the team leader?

5. *The impact of external pressures*
   - Is the team able to do its work?
   - Are the goals of the organization overwhelming the ability of the team to address them?
   - Is the number of issues in the agenda sufficient to ensure team success?
   - Is the team clear about its contribution and role in decision making in the system?

- Does the system provide sufficient supports to the team to facilitate the team's work?
- Is the system's atmosphere one that supports team-based activity and decision making?
- Do decisions occurring outside the team confuse the locus of control and the authority of the team to make its decisions?
- Does system leadership appear to support the activities of the team and facilitate its interdependence and independence in decision making?
- Is the team's development, learning and advancement encouraged and facilitated by systems leadership to ensure its effectiveness?

TOOL E: Responses to Getting Unstuck: A Checklist

1. *Review the team's purpose.* Periodically it is wise to reaffirm and reassert the purpose of the team to ensure that team members are aware of it and act consistent with it. The purpose of the team drives the functions of team members and therefore should be clear, identifiable, and understandable by team members at all times during the team's work. Often as the team gets mired in its business, its purpose gets lost. Revisiting the purpose of the team and its basic formation principles helps reaffirm and reassert those foundations for the team's activities and its success.

2. *Ensure the team's viability.* Sometimes the teams are initiated with the expectation for performance without sufficient information or authority. Teams cannot be sustainable unless they have the right resources and the authority to do their work. Therefore reviewing the

foundations of the team, the decision-making framework for the team, and the range of expectations and activities directed to the team is a critical element for team success.

3. *Ensure appropriate information support.* Often there are questions around the team's ability to have the resources necessary to do its required work. Therefore review of the information, services, supports, and systems available to it helps team members be clear about what access they have to the resources they need to make good decisions. Information is critical to the success of the work of the team. Therefore its relationship to the information support structure is important to its viability. Being clear about its information needs and accessed information helps break some of the barriers around the team's long-term effectiveness.

4. *Build successes as you go.* Aggregated success depends on the number of small successes that can be enumerated as a team does its work. Identifying these small successes and naming them becomes a critical mechanism for measuring team effectiveness and maintaining the team's enthusiasm. Being able to succeed creates more motivation for further success. Enumerating those successes and building on them creates an energy level that sustains the activity in the work of the team over the long term.

5. *Facilitate leadership.* The leadership must be capable of providing good facilitation and direction for the team. Using good process discipline, techniques, methods and processes is critical to team leadership effectiveness. When the team is not able to use good process, the members lose faith and confidence in team leadership. Leadership skill, energy commitment, and competence of the leader are important variables for sustaining the energy and effectiveness of the team and are critical to the ability of the team to maintain the energy necessary to do its work.

6. *Ensure an effective transition of team members.* When members are unable to perform, to act consistently, to meet expectations, or to relate with other members, questions regarding their continuing membership are appropriate. If individuals and leaders on a team cannot perform consistent with the expectations and give evidence of their unwillingness to do so, changes in members and leaders must be considered. A team must be effective to sustain the system's work and the outcomes of the organization. Leadership always has a dramatic impact on the effectiveness and sustainability of the team. When that needs to change the team must take action quickly.

TOOLF: Comprehensive Team Readiness Assessment

The environment for building teams is as important as the skills in constructing teams themselves. Questions around the ability of the team to function and operate effectively are critical to the sustenance of the team. All of these elements affecting team performance are important considerations in ensuring the long-term effectiveness of team actions.

Instructions: Use the following questions and issues to serve as a checklist to determine whether all of the elements affecting the sustainability of teams have been considered by the team leadership:

1. *Size*
   - Is it convenient to get the team members together in one place?
   - Can the team members relate to each other in a direct and meaningful way?
   - Can the discussions be open, free flowing, and frank?
   - Can discussion around roles, skill, ability, talent, and application be held easily in a free-flowing manner?
   - Are the right people in the room?

- Is there appropriate diversity and distribution of representative membership to be able to do the business of the team?
2. *Team competence*
   - Are those representing the disciplines or the work of the organization clearly able to make that representation?
   - Do the people in the room have the functional, conceptual, and application talents necessary to contribute to the discussion?
   - Are the people in the room able to enter into the relationships and interactions necessary for high-intensity dialogue at the team level?
   - Are the critical thinking processes necessary to deliberate successfully present in the membership in the room?
   - Do those in the room express their commitment to the work and activities that will be undertaken there?
3. *Meaning*
   - Are the mission and purpose of the meeting and the team clear to each member?
   - Can each member identify the direction of the team and its value and work as it undertakes its activities?
   - Is there a high level of general energy and commitment in the room around the issues and functions of the team?
   - Is there a level of enthusiasm and excitement around the issues, processes, and authorities expressed within the context of the team?
4. *Outcomes*
   - Is every member of the team oriented toward the achievement of outcomes?
   - Is there a straightforward relationship between the critical processes identified and the outcomes to which they are directed?

- Are all team members able to articulate their contribution to outcome?
- Is the outcome delineated realistic, appropriate, and within the functional capacity of the team?
- Do all team members recognize the importance of specific outcomes in relationship to their own work and the team's collective action?
- Do all members of the team agree on the specific outcomes and the processes directed toward them?
5. *Work*
   - Are team members aware of the work they must do to facilitate the outcomes of the team?
   - Does each team member have specific work, functions, and capacity that have been articulated and identified?
   - Does each team member feel equal contribution to the work of the team and participation in the team's process?
   - Are the dynamics of the dialogue balanced, effective, and inclusive?
   - Do members indicate a clear understanding of the learning process associated with their application of skill within the team format?

The above elements identify the contextual framework for the function of a team. Every team has its own characteristics, personality, and culture. However, to operate effectively each team must be able to address the above items consistently over the life of the team. A deficit in any of the above items generally creates a need for the team to stop progress and work and to deliberate its response to the deficit area.

8

Trust: A Prerequisite for Sustaining a Team-Based System

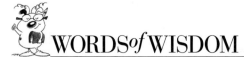

WORDS*of*WISDOM

Believe no one who claims to have the right answer . . . it is only a sign of ignorance or self-interest.

⌒

Recently, a company name Allied Signal recognized that to stay competitive, it had to retool its organization from a culture of control and manipulation to one that really motivated workers. It implemented a team-based system because it understood that success would come when employees understood their jobs from the perspective of the whole product, not simply their particular job. As the result of shifting to teams, 99.8% of the products shipped in 1996 were sent on the required date. In the mid-1980s, the number of products shipped on time was only 8.9% (Lilley, 1996).

Today more than ever the antecedents of success for the health care enterprise depend on the cooperation of all staff members, who either work in direct care or support the care delivery at the point of service. Simply stated, doubtful or distrustful staff members do not cooperate in the attainment of organizational goals, no matter how noble. Employee distrust is growing in the face of downsizing, mergers, and rapid change. It is expressed in several subtle and not so subtle behaviors (Box 8-1).

BOX 8-1

The Impact of Employee Distrust

- The degree of involvement or abdication in the improvement of working methods and procedures
- The accuracy of operations reporting, based on truthful estimations of workload
- The rate at which mistakes are detected early and the number of interventions when mistakes do occur
- The achievement of team consensus on the behaviors of professional integrity, sincerity, mutual trust, and unconditional commitment to definitions of the team's work
- The acceptance of accountability for action or nonaction

TEAM TRUST-BUSTERS

Teams are very much influenced by the issue of trust. The ability to build commitment, attachment, and mutual trust significantly influences how well teams perform their accountabilities. There are eight team "trust-busters" that will foster the development of dysfunctional and therefore ineffective teams.

Disbelief in Procedural Justice*

In this situation, there is a lack of procedural justice, coloring team members' belief in fairness. It comes from unfair work procedures employed by the team and fostered by its leaders. Team members believe that there are inequitable opportunities to provide input and influence. The experience of what is perceived to be biased work procedures diminishes not only

---

*Kossgard MA, Schweiger DM, Sappienze, HJ: Building commitment, attachment, and trust in strategic decision making teams: the role of procedural justice, *Academy of Management Journal* 38(1):60-85, 1995.

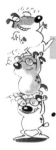

TEAM**TIP**   8.1

Antidotes for Procedural Injustice

- *Regularly review the team's process of working together. Make this a normative process for the team by setting aside team meetings periodically to evaluate performance.*
- *Use the open-ended questionnaire, Evaluating Your Team's Work Processes, found at the end of this chapter, to ensure the objective evaluation of assumptions and experiences.*
- *Use an outside facilitator if you have determined that the team leader or manager share accountability for unfair work processes.*

members' commitment to the group's decision, but also their attachment to the group and their trust in leaders. Team Tip 8-1 give antidotes for procedural injustice.

For example, a quality improvement team was chaired by the department's quality improvement director. She had her own agendas, related to her recent poor performance appraisal. She used the team to do her work, therefore improving her performance. When team members complained that they were not following their team charter nor were they allowed to disagree with the "decisions" made by the team, they were told by the leader that regulations required the work to be performed in the way she was directing them to do it. The team was eventually disbanded because it did not meet its original charter and was deemed redundant. The quality director was promoted, and decentralized quality work became a thing of the past.

Poor Cooperation of Team Members in Fully Sharing Information

When each team member shares his or her knowledge and experience, there is added value to the team's decisions. Members have plentiful opportunities to cooperate fully in the sharing of helpful information and experiences. In turn, this cooperation makes it likely that each person can fully support the team's final decision. When trust is absent, there is no commitment to the execution of the team's decisions. People will stall implementation efforts or actually sabotage them. You know you have poor cooperation in fully sharing either personal reactions or expert opinions when:

1. People nod their heads or are silent in response to a statement or question. This false consensus signals fear of sharing an opposite viewpoint and hesitancy to engage in healthy dialogue.
2. People who question information or request more information are labeled as "non-team players" who are obstructing the team from getting its work done.

3. Language games such as the use of jargon, misstating facts, or burying members under complex, unreadable reports are common.

Team Tip 8-2 gives antidotes for inadequate information.

Alienation Within the Team Is Allowed to Flourish

Attachment to the team unfolds as team members get to know one another, feel part of the team, and look forward to working together. When alienation is allowed to flourish, people never come to that special fellowship of a committed team. Instead, team members continue to pursue their individual self-interests at the expense of the team. This limits team flexibility, particularly in evaluating multiple options and differences in opinions.

For example, alienation is unwittingly fostered by allowing the work of the team to be seen as something less important than patient care. In

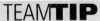

TEAM**TIP**   8.2

Antidotes for Inadequate Information

It is essential that in the Team Accountability Contract (see Chapter 4) there is documentation that the team accepts and welcomes challenges in the process of reaching consensus.

Continually reinforce that decisions need to be data driven. Ask questions such as "Do we have all of the information that we need?" and "Is this decision truly data driven?" Always apply the three C's to any information collected or presented to the team: is it current, complete, and certain?

BOX **8-2**

Example from the Field

A newly formed management team was having trouble making consensus decisions and was performing at a mediocre level. It seemed that a recent management restructuring had significantly altered the membership of this decision-making group. Members were now from different departments, different reporting structures, and different types of management positions. Because the organization remained traditionally structured, they rarely ran into each other in the course of their daily work. Because they did not know one another very well as people, they were hesitant to trust each other in the conduct of the real dialogue necessary for consensus building.

fact, the work of teams must contribute to the enhancement of patient care. When teamwork is seen as something "extra" by managers, there is inadequate support for team members to be "freed" from patient care to do the work of the team. When several members are absent at every meeting, teams fail to develop, opportunism flourishes, and eventually the team disbands.

Emotional distance between team members also reduces the ability of team members to trust each other and live with differences in their individual perspectives. It also allows some team members to be more productive than others, resulting in an uneven workload and resentment. Box 8-2 gives an example of alienation within the team. Team Tip 8-3 gives antidotes for alienation.

TEAM**TIP**   8.3

Antidotes for Alienation

- *Develop a competency-based job description for the team leader role. Team members must have faith in the honesty, goodwill, and sincerity of the team leader, if they are to become attached to the team.*
- *Do the same for the advisor role. If team members do not believe that they can work in an atmosphere of mutual trust, they will avoid participation and the interpersonal connection necessary for success.*
- *Never charter a team unless the team's work is truly tied to the patient care outcomes required by the organization. Hold managers accountable for articulating the value of the team's contributions to patient care.*
- *Challenge personal agendas.*

Misguided Intent*

In health care organizations, where the specialization of interest flourishes, misguided intent is epidemic. Harm is caused unintentionally through ignorance, duress, or the rationalization of events. Heartless actions may be taken that are "strictly a business decision" or rationalized as "simply doing our jobs." Consider the following example. A new surgical nurse caught herself making a medication error. She had begun to add the wrong antibiotic to a patient's intravenous line, but caught herself before any of the medication was administered. The nurse documented the incident, met with her manager, and received a verbal warning. The manager knew her well, trusted her work, and saw the high level of commitment she had to her patients. She felt a reprimand was in order but also coached the nurse on time management and priority setting.

In this particular organization, incident reports are automated and recorded in the risk management department. On the Monday morning after the incident, this same manager was directed by the vice-president of risk management to suspend the nurse because he, the vice-president of risk management, had come from a hospital that was "soft on patient safety," and he would "not tolerate that developing in this organization." His position put the manager in a no-win situation and was totally ignorant of the human side of the incident.

Misguided intent is a trust-buster because it appears as indifference. Ethical issues are never discussed. People relinquish personal accountability for tough, ethical decisions. Eventually a form of cognitive dissonance grows among employees when what is right conflicts that what is actually happening.

In another example from the field, the management structure was flattened and new, combined, and more accountable manager roles were developed by the organization. Unfortunately in the implementation, the

*Colero L: Common sense ethics in business, *World Business Academy Perspectives* 9(1):67-75, 1995.

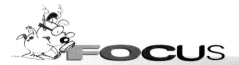

FOCUS

Team Leader/Advisor Competencies

- Eases team through processes to achieve goals
- Recognizes outcomes are based on work of members
- Is a positive force in implementation
- Facilitates positive team dynamics
- Assists team to integrate ideal with reality
- Identifies operational implications to team decision making
- Consistently shares emerging organization issues with the team
- Accepts inevitability of politics and assists teams to respond effectively
- Facilitates team learning
- Challenges the quality of information

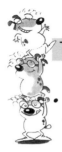

TEAM**TIP**   8.4

Antidotes to Misguided Intent

- *Watch for symptoms of organizational groupthink: honest belief that the unethical action is the right thing to do and ignorance of its impact.*
- *Know when to use a process for the impartial delineation of the facts, such as a cost-benefit analysis or risk analysis.*
- *Avoid knee-jerk decisions that offer quick solutions but sidetrack into faulty decisions. Allow time for reflection about what the right thing is to do in this instance.*
- *Be a model for candor and integrity.*
- *Ask yourself, "How would I feel if this action was described in the next issue of Hospitals and Health Networks?"*
- *Support those who honestly challenge intent.*

tough decisions of competence were not addressed. Seniority-strong but incompetent managers were put into the new roles. People became increasingly uncomfortable with this disharmony and found the consequences too hard to think about, much less discuss. Peer pressure grew, encouraging people to remain blind, not saying aloud what they actually were seeing. It became more and more difficult for people to trust anyone about any kind of change being proposed in this organization. Team Tip 8-4 features antidotes to misguided intent.

Managing People with Paternalism/Maternalism*

The nurturing, caring nature of health care service is sometimes its own worst enemy, because these features so essential to good patient outcomes can be a disaster when they become the predominant management style. When people are managed like children, they make choices out of guilt or acquiescence. The consequences of acting or not acting are defined by

---

*Hanson R: An analysis of the concept of mutuality, *Image: The Journal of Nursing Scholarship* 29(1):39-45, 1997.

TEAM**TIP**   8.5

Antidotes to Parental Management Styles

- *Replace paternalism/maternalism with mutuality.*
- *Insist on the team outcomes of mutuality.*
- *Watch for and recognize gestures, looks, language, and actions that foster mutuality. Use these examples to teach others the signs of mutual relationships.*
- *Understand how your own "parent messages," developed in your own family, play out in your management style . . . both the nurturing and the critical messages.*

powerful others. So, why not park your brains at the door when you come to work? A mind is indeed a terrible thing to waste. Patients, families, co-workers, and the organization are the losers in this instance. People managed in this way are robbed of the opportunity to trust their own judgments and to become more self-managing. Team Tip 8-5 features antidotes to parental management styles.

Language Games*

Language shapes organizational events. Articulate leaders can compress the scope of employee thinking so that people cannot think dissident thoughts. Formal definitions can be used to define words into their opposites. For example, too much freedom in shared leadership groups is seen as a negative because it is defined as a form of slavery to the group.

Doublespeak is another language game. The communicator deliberately clouds the message in a pretense of communicating. Some people are masters at making the bad appear good or applying euphemisms to avoid harsh realities.

Jargon, or the specialized language applied by a professional group as a form of shorthand, can be used to obsfucate rather than to illuminate. Have you ever sat down with a computer programmer to get to the bottom of a problem with a report that you needed, and found yourself completely baffled by the discussion? Have you found, with the merging of patient care units or functional departments, that enormous communication problems are the source of seemingly endless issues with the change? Chances are, jargon is getting in the way.

When manipulative definitions, doublespeak, or jargon is used in communicating with teams, credibility and trust in the message is not possible. People sit and listen, wondering what the communicator is really trying to say. Because teams are heavily reliant on the character of

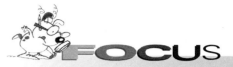

FOCUS

Outcomes of Mutuality

- *Increased sense of situational control*
- *Increased ability to engage in self-management*
- *Satisfaction with relationship*
- *Optimized creativity*

*Mohr WK: The outcomes of corporate greed, *Image: The Journal of Nursing Scholarship* 29(1):39-45, 1997.

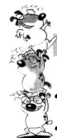

TEAM**TIP**   8.6

Antidotes to Language Games

- *Develop ground rules that protect people who report language games.*
- *Ensure that everyone is held to a social contract with each other, to communicate in a clear, comprehensive, well-intentioned manner.*
- *Model the positive confrontation of people using language games. Staff members spend a fair amount of time watching manager behavior. This is the quickest way to develop an organizational norm.*
- *Never assume that the other party understands you. Check in with your listeners, asking questions such as "Am I making any sense here?" This type of question invites people to admit their confusion.*
- *Keep good minutes. Never allow poorly worded or inaccurate descriptions to go uncorrected. This only perpetuates miscommunication. Really read minutes before approving them, rather than the all too typical once-over glance and quick approval.*
- *Always try to be sensitive to the other party's point of view. If you can address the unique perspective of other parties in your communication, you create the foundation for more dialogue.*

the information they receive, the quality of their decisions will be affected by language games, particularly in the case of purposeful confusion or manipulation. Team Tip 8-6 features antidotes to language games. Unfortunately, language games are one of the most popular strategies used by those who want to see teams fail. The sad news is that they almost always work.

Putting People in No-Win Situations

When team members or their leaders are put in no-win situations, they withdraw from the situation and fail to take action on otherwise actionable issues. For example, people in one organization were asked to look the other way when a carefully negotiated problem-solving process in the new team-based system was ignored, so that the old bureaucracy could prevail. No-win situations are also created when powerful others publicly misstate the facts of a situation. This can happen when a leader fails to understand just what the work of the team was and how the situation came into existence. In this case, teams feel devalued and distrustful of executive support.

Shifting blame to another person or department and telling people to cover mistakes are also very potent ways to put people in no-win situations. A common example is the nursing director who tells her staff members that "absolutely nothing is to leave this department." This makes it almost impossible for the staff members from this department to participate in multidisciplinary teams with any semblance of honesty. Team Tip 8-7 gives antidotes to no-win situations.

Employ Systems of Blame Instead of Systems of Accountability*

Although significant lip service is given to accountability, the truth is that it is woefully absent in many organizations. When there are no accountability systems, there has to be a mechanism for problem solving. The process that replaces accountability is blame. Something goes wrong, there is a search for the responsible party, the culprits are named and punished, so the problem goes away. The burden is shifted and a short-term fix is once again in place. Blame is also an excellent strategy for

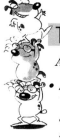

TEAMTIP   8.7

Antidotes to No-Win Situations

- Always listen to the other side. You may not realize how your approach affects the other person's actions.
- Ask for and encourage feedback. Avoid defensive responses.
- Be careful not to fall into that old "blame game": If it were not for you, I (we) would have . . . Take accountability only for that which you have contributed to a circumstance, and encourage others to do the same.

---

*Paul MC: Moving from blame to accountability: *The Systems Thinker* 8(1):1-6, 1997.

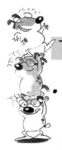

TEAM**TIP**   8.8

Antidotes to Blame

- *Provide behavioral learning experiences that are designed to challenge and change how people think about blame.*
- *Clarify accountabilities in advance through clear contracting of each party, dialogue, and organizational commitment to support accountability over blame.*
- *Remind yourself that anger, judgment, and criticism prevent effective problem solving. Work constructively with these feelings either before or while actually making decisions.*
- *Work to understand the organizational pressures that are affecting each party in the situation. Sometimes a person's or a team's performance is the result of something unknown to you. Perhaps they are working on an impossible job or do not have enough resources to perform well.*

avoiding focus on long-term solutions to structural or interpersonal issues. Or is it? Blame costs the organization, because people are fearful of standing up and owning what they may have contributed to a situation. Instead, they are tied up in the emotions of the situation. Team Tip 8-8 gives antidotes to blame.

THE CREATION OF A HUMANE WORKPLACE

For many of us, the slogan "Give Peace a Chance" reminds us of our all too recent past and the great divisions that split our country during the Vietnam War. The brutality of war was something everyone could agree on, although individual positions on the Vietnam War varied from zero tolerance to zealous militarism. Now it is our workplaces that are at times very brutal. The manager in a team-based organization must actively work to ensure that peace is in the workplace, by acknowledging and supporting people's humanity.

In South Africa, the term *Ubuntu* is a new management theory term that, translated from Zulu, means "I can only be me through your eyes." It comes from the phrase "A human is a human because of other people." This holds true for the manager as well. Social science and management theories have taken only a part of leadership and substituted it for the whole . . . neglecting a significant portion of what makes us humans and what it means to be human (Bolman and Deal, 1995). Soul, spirit, and the heart of a person at work are central to the meaningful and successful enactment of relationship-centered management. In the health care workplace, we all need a language of moral discourse that permits discussions of ethical, spiritual, cognitive, and psychological issues, connecting them to images of leadership. The absence of a common language does not permit us to truly discuss the humane issues we face in either our operational decision making or our care delivery. There is a kind of taboo associated with talking of spiritual matters or matters of the heart in the workplace. This robs people of their courage and conviction to do what they believe to be right (Whyte, 1994).

Consider some of the track records of contemporary health care organizations. Do any of these examples sound familiar? Layoffs of clinical staff members are employed every time there is red ink, rather than facing the difficult corporate system and behavioral issues. Critical decisions are postponed because of leader uncertainty, causing massive anxiety and low morale. Months of work by chartered work teams are tossed aside, with little understanding of the effort involved. Some managers are dishonest with caregivers, calling downsizing efforts work redesign. Others publicly support change but in private or in small groups predict dire outcomes . . . and then wonder why there is so much anger and militancy in the organization.

Our traditional models of leadership have failed to solve the deepening self-esteem problems of the health care workplace. Organizations are scrambling to downsize in the hope of avoiding extinction. Frazzled and exhausted managers scratch their heads, confronted with new problems for which there are no clear answers. Staff members suffer because, in the midst of confusion, many management groups are simply surfing from one new management fad to another. We lost our way when we forgot that the heart of leadership lies in the hearts and souls of leaders. We fooled ourselves into believing that flow charts could respond to our deepest concerns. To recapture our humanity we need to learn how to lead with our soul and create community.

Soul and spirit are defined differently. *Soul* is personal and unique, grounded in the depths of your human experience. *Spirit,* on the other hand, is that special community of an organization filled with people who embrace shared values, goals, and vision (Moore, 1991). Managers with soul bring humanity into the health care workplace.

The relationship-centered manager works to leave behind the mechanistic mental models of the past and instead creates a humane workplace with four kinds of relationships: care, power, ownership, and significance.

WORDS *of* WISDOM

Be careful to avoid becoming personally involved, you might just forget the organization's interpretation of this event.

QUESTIONS OF CARE

How do you express passion in your organization? How do people know you care? We have been taught as managers to remain objective at the price of authentic relationships. The price we have paid for adopting this practice is large human resource departments whose job is to tell you what the staff members are thinking and feeling. Do you know if your followers care about you? Care is contagious. Care cannot only be expressed once a year during hospital week or at Christmas when managers serve employees meals.

Care is expressed in the act of being fully present on a day-to-day basis. What do you do that signals your devotion to the growth and development of your teams?

When you have to take a layoff action, do you personally talk to those who have been laid off? The lesson to be learned is that you get what you give. Many contemporary managers have not even recognized that they have already lost something! The potential of teams is diminished when managers fail to create work relationships grounded in caring and compassion.

QUESTIONS OF POWER

We have to let go of the misconception that management is expressed through individual heroism. Unfortunately, the individual pursuit of heroism is alive and well in the ranks of health care management. Some managers compete with one another to see who is the best hero, who is the best wager of war, who is the best champion of great causes, or who is the hero for single-handedly changing the course of an organization—this month! With heroism comes a certain amount of influence and power. The question of course is whether the heroism is enacted for the benefit of those we serve or for the pursuit of one's own career agenda.

Consider the nurse executive whose major career goal was to be accepted into the American Academy of Nursing. Any innovation she chose to adopt was carefully selected with that goal in mind, rather than the needs of those she served in her administrative capacity. You can easily tell if this phenomenon is operational in your own organization. The self-serving hero rarely has the stamina to see an innovation all the way to completion, often moving on to a "greater career opportunity" when transformation becomes challenging.

Another archetypal hero common to health care is the autonomous lonely Superwoman, living on the fringe of society. People who emulate this hero model of leadership often pay a heavy personal price: alienation, feelings of failure, stress-related illness, and even early death. They create situations where their teams have unmitigated loyalty to the leader, even when the leader is embarked in the wrong direction. Team members are robbed of a sense of their own competence. Teams never experience the influence that can be derived from their achievements, because they live in the shadow of their hero.

Team-based organization must operate in the context of community and shared power. Hero-managers do not create this environment. Building community means that successful managers embody their teams' most precious values and beliefs. Managers' ability to lead will emerge from the strengths and sustenance of those around them. You must be able to engage in relationship-building activities that help both individuals and teams to develop the capacity for their own heroism.

Stripping people of their power results in a powerless organization where people simply look for ways to fight back, sabotage, withdraw, or engage in militancy. When power is hoarded, conflict is often suppressed, and when it does emerge it is in coercive or explosive forms. Team-based organizations find more productive ways to handle conflict. Sharing power always creates difficult choice points and struggle with letting go or holding the reins too tightly. Team-based systems demand that conflict be resolved without physical or emotional bloodshed, but with grace and dignity. It begins with managers themselves.

QUESTIONS OF OWNERSHIP

How do you act when you feel that you have influence? Do you create those conditions for others? Can you recognize that managers rob people

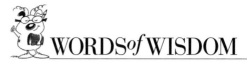

WORDS*of*WISDOM

The definition of a superhero is a person we created to let ourselves off the hook.

of influence when they allow upward delegation or when they accept those things that the staff members can solve themselves as management problems? Can you admit the fact that as managers, we love being the people who solve the tough problems?

The outcome? We let people off the hook, protecting them from making mistakes and learning. Meanwhile, we rarely have time to see the big picture because we are so swamped in daily problem solving. In Japan, it is the group's job to solve the problem of the leader (Bolman and Deal, 1995).

It is up to you to break the cycle of control and taking credit for the hard work of others. This is none other than a subtle way of hoarding power . . . not as blatant as flaming oppression but just as powerful.

Managers in team-based systems create the opportunities for people to put their own signature in their work. This stimulates the sheer human joy of providing a service of lasting value and adding something of value to the delivery of care. People need to see their work as meaningful and worthwhile, to feel personally accountable for the consequence of their efforts, and to get feedback that tells them the results of their action.

Ownership begins with autonomy and power. One cannot own without the ability to influence outcomes. They need each other, in that both are only meaningful in relationship to others. Power without authorship is destructive, and authorship without influence is meaningless (Bolman and Deal, 1995).

QUESTIONS OF SIGNIFICANCE

What are the times when you felt significant? How did people mark the special moments in your life? Maybe what works for you will work in your organization. You cannot impose significance; it has to be created together. Significance comes from working with others to do something worthwhile.

How much of the work performed by people in your organizations is experienced by them to be insignificant? For people to experience significance, the organization has to be *ours,* not mine. Can you think of a time in your organization when as a whole, you felt the significance of accomplishment? Maybe it was a successful accreditation survey. Perhaps it was the formal ceremony signaling the passing of the torch from management to teams or the resolution of a particularly difficult situation. In team-based organizations, the manager is challenged to make significance a part of the health care work experience. Rituals, stories, ceremonies, or T-shirts can build significance. They must be authentic, shared, and able to fire the imagination and heart. These symbols, rooted in real values, cannot be allowed to disappear in times of crisis. Box 8-3 provides an example of significance run amuck.

THROUGH THE LOOKING GLASS

The key to new forms of managing begins with your own personal work. In our experience, the failure to truly transform ourselves and our organizations lies in managers' lack of willingness to look in the mirror and to see both the beauty and the beast . . . and to act on what is authentically seen.

To act on the creation of a humane workplace means to examine your relationships in the context of caring, ownership, power, and significance. Determine how these human experiences affect the people where you practice. The next step is to eliminate those that are barriers to an authentic team-based workplace.

Managers in team-based organizations have no authority except that which comes from wisdom, competence, experience, and relationships. They know that in times of difficulty, teams must try to learn again. These leaders provide the nucleus on which teams develop and grow. Leaders who will share their humanity with us if we ask them . . . leaders who love.

BOX **8-3**

> ### *Example from the Field*
>
> A certain company began its reengineering efforts by surveying its employees. Based on survey feedback, they made certain changes, including upgrading the toilet paper in the employee bathrooms and establishing casual dress days on Fridays. In the next phase of the project, they eliminated 5000 jobs! An enterprising group of remaining employees created and wore T-shirts that read: "Two-ply. No Tie. Good-Bye."

Bibliography

Bolman LG, Deal TE: *Leading with soul,* San Francisco, Jossey-Bass, 1995.

Colero L: Common sense ethics in business, *World Business Academy Perspectives* 9(1):67-75, 1995.

Dauten D: Satisfying customers, not reengineering is the key, *Arizona Republic Newspapers,* October 28, 1996, E-4.

Hanson R: An analysis of the concept of mutuality, *Image: The Journal of Nursing Scholarship* 29(1):39-45, 1997.

Kossgard MA, Schweiger DM, Sapienza HJ: Building commitment, attachment and trust in strategic decision making teams: the role of procedural justice, *Academy of Management Journal* 38(1):60-85, 1995.

Lilley V: Thriving business culture depends upon trust, *The Kansas City Business Journal,* May 17, 1996.

Mohr WK: The outcomes of corporate greed, *Image: The Journal of Nursing Scholarship* 29(1):45-52, 1997.

Moore T: *Blue fire: selected writings by James Hillman,* New York, HarperCollins, 1991.

Paul MC: Moving from blame to accountability, *The Systems Thinker* 8(1):1-6, 1997.

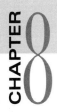

TOOLCHEST

TOOL A: Evaluating Your Team's Work Processes

Instructions: Select one of the most recent decisions made by your team. Have each member make an assessment of the decision and the degree to which he or she feels committed to it. Next, openly review the team's accountability contract. Instruct each member to privately complete his or her own assessment of the team's performance, answering the questions below. Ask members to privately compare each member's earlier assumptions and commitment to the selected decision with their own before answering each question. The leader or outside facilitator then leads the team in a discussion of each member's responses to the items, looking for commonalities and differences with the team's work processes. Work to come to consensus on work processes that everyone can agree are fair.

1. How satisfied are you with your team's most recent decision?
2. To what extent does the plan reflect the ideas and viewpoints of all of the members?
3. What process did you use to arrive at the plan and to determine which ideas to incorporate and which to exclude?
4. How satisfied are you with this process? Which elements of the process pleased you? Which displeased you?
5. How did the process fit with the team's accountability guidelines, developed by all of you when you first came together as a team?
6. Did everyone participate in the discussion? If so, how did the group achieve total participation? If not, what inhibited the participation of some members?
7. What member behaviors helped support group work?
8. What behaviors hindered group work?
9. As you worked together, how did you handle conflict?
10. How did this activity reflect the way in which you typically work together? What atypical behaviors arose? How can you use this information in your work together in the future?
11. What are the benefits of working together in your particular team to solve problems? What can you do to ensure that your collective expertise is applied in future team efforts at problem solving?
12. What are the drawbacks to team efforts? How can you help overcome some of these drawbacks?
13. Did you have the information you needed to make decisions? What was the quality of that information?

TOOL B: Trust Dialogue

Instructions: The list of questions below is designed to stimulate team discussions of trust-related topics. Each team member takes a few minutes to ask a question. Going around the group, each member responds to the question. Once feedback has been obtained from every member, including the person asking the question, the team evaluates itself for trust-busting activities. Questions to be asked and answered include the following: Is there a team trust issue that we can identify from the discussion of this question? If so, what do we need to do? The following ground rules should be applied when engaged in this dialogue:

- Take turns in asking questions to the team as a whole. Each team member must select a question to ask of the team.
- Each member must participate in answering the question that he or she asks.
- Use active listening, paraphrasing, and summarizing skills to ensure that you understand what each person is communicating.
- Before beginning this dialogue, review expectations of confidentiality.

Questions of Trust

1. What do we think the next step is in our team's development?

2. How do we feel about ourselves as members of this team?
3. Are there any personal temperaments of team members that are getting in the way of the team's work? If so, how can we deal with these?
4. How do you perceive of me as a member of this team?
5. What would you predict to be my assessment of each of you?
6. What kind of relationship does each of us want with our team?
7. What factors in your job situation impede your ability to contribute to this team?
8. Are there certain group members with whom you have the most difficulty in understanding their perspective? What is it about that point of view? How do you react?
9. On a scale of 1 to 10 (with 10 being full commitment and 1 being no commitment), how committed are you to the work of this team?
10. What role do you play in this team?
11. How do you want to receive feedback from this team?
12. What issues do you think the team must face together?

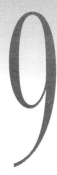

Functioning in an Effective Team

WHY CHARTER YOUR TEAM?

To charter a team means to create a mental model for success. The chartering methodology is often underestimated or completely overlooked because managers do not recognize its value to team performance. As the team charter is created and implemented, certain critical outcomes are achieved:

- Through purposeful action steps, a clear model for team success is established.
- A road map to effective performance is created, amplifying the team's contributions to organizational goals. The work of any team must also be congruent with the strategic and the value structure of the organization.
- Because team-based systems are cross-functional in nature, the essential functions for each team are delineated along with the outcomes of those functions.
- The organization defines and then supports the acquisition of appropriate competencies for successful teamwork, along with tools and processes to apply them.

- New expectations for individual and team performance are established, along with the tools to monitor and evaluate their realization.
- The accounting of team outcomes measures ensures that the team contributes to organizational goals and provides for intervention in mediocre performance.

Health care team development is distinct because all multidisciplinary functions must be aligned with the methods of the care delivery system. These include service planning and delivery, innovation execution, error reduction and problem solving, outcomes achievement, variance analysis, and performance monitoring. When health care teams and their functions are so aligned, the delivery of patient care services becomes more timely, of better quality, and more cost-effective. If structured well, team-based systems can reduce the time it takes to implement new services, from 3 to 5 years to 1 year (Taincez, 1996).

WHAT IF YOU DECIDE TO SKIP THE WORK OF CHARTERING YOUR TEAMS?

- There will be consequences that will limit your success.
- Staff who have been working in your organization for a long time are usually quite comfortable in their roles and functions. Team-based systems require that they leave the comfort of a predictable specialty niche. This is not a simple process.
- Managers and staff alike will move only if they see the ramifications and risks that accompany staying in their technical worlds. They must be able to articulate not only how patient care will benefit from a new way of working together but also the ramification of failing to personally acquire team skills.
- This cannot be achieved without the implementation of a chartering methodology.

CHARTERING TEAMS: CREATING A TEAM MENTAL MODEL

- An individual mental model is essentially a psychological representation of the environment and expected behaviors. Its purpose is to assist human beings in the work of cognitive processing, by providing a shortcut that describes, explains, and predicts future states.
- Mental models allow people to screen out unnecessary information, limit information overload, and reduce intolerable anxiety resulting from confusion.
- A team mental model is the shared cognition of a group of people. It is developed through creation of a team charter and reinforced through repeated application as the team performs its work. Group affect, collective effectiveness, problem solving, membership factors and the quality of interpersonal relationships are social processes influenced by team charters.
- The work of chartering a team is the cornerstone of a carefully negotiated thought structure that transcends the individual belief systems.
- A team mental model provides the script for team action. Well-developed teams have an observable pattern of behaviors that allow them to perform well. Role expectations, team norms, behavioral routines, and clear expectations about how team members should behave in certain situations are imbedded in the procedural knowledge of a team mental model (Klimoski and Mohammed, 1994).

CHARTERING YOUR TEAM (SEE TEAM CHARTER TOOL CHEST)

Create a Team Mission Statement

Before you begin, be clear about what the creation of a mission statement will actually do for a team. Far too many people have sat through mindless planning sessions to create strategic plans or mission statements, only to see their work collect dust on a shelf. Document the reasons for moving

Remember that a team's shared vision is really the team norms. As different types of work issues confront the team for action, leaders will need to recognize that there may be as many mental models as there are members about that particular issue. Do not try to reach a "shared vision" in such instances. Instead work to consensus, recognizing the rich diversity of viewpoints.

Team mental models contain the shared expectations of the tasks and the authority of the team. They allow teams to more accurately predict what behaviors are needed to complete a task and to quickly identify resources needed for outcome achievement.

to a team-based system, who the team is, what the team does, and how individual mission supports organizational goal achievement. This may be different for different teams. A team mission statement helps people connect with what the team is and provides guidelines for daily decision making. A clear mission statement helps teams to know what to do when confronted with unexpected situations. Team-based systems demand that people exert individual behavior control rather than management control. A carefully worded mission statement can help teams to know how to behave. The mission statement should be short, concise, and motivating. It should paint a clear picture of the future and the team's accountability in getting there. Describe the team's external focus. Who are the team's customers? What are the team's critical network relationships? What does the team do for its customers? Describe the team's internal focus (Emery, 1996).

- What are the team's core values? What underlying values are important for team performance? For example, if teams are multidisciplinary and multifunctional in membership, diversity of viewpoints is very important to team performance.
- What unique talents are represented on the team? How is this team different than others? What is the unique contribution of this team to organizational goals?

Roles and Definitions

The team charter assists with the work of transformation. People will need assistance in feeling positive about a newly reorganized work environment. In the change process, it is not always clear what the benefits are to anyone. Team charters provide clear reminders of why the environment must change. Define the accountabilities of each member, including team leaders, facilitators, advisors, functional specialists, and team members in general. What do team member accountabilities look like? Samples of a redesign project team leader, executive advisor, and specialized team roles are located at the end of this chapter. These are useful handouts to accompany a team charter workshop. Define how the team relates to the organizational structure. Where does the team fit? What can be expected from teams? What are the boundaries of team authority? Organizational members need this information to work in a team-based system. Delineate new processes critical to team performance: alterations in information flow to include teams, new communication systems, and new feedback loops.

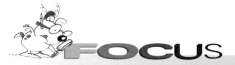

FOCUS

Potential Team Roles

- Leader
- Management advisor
- Functional specialists
- Quality improvement
- Risk management
- Finance/human resources
- Individual team members
- Executive coach

Integrate the Team-Based System and Strategic Plan

Carefully articulate the reasons why you believe a team-based system will get you where you want to be. Document precisely what the team-based system provides in terms of added value to the accomplishment of organizational goals. *Note:* This item defines the team-based system contribution to organizational goals. Individual team contributions are included in the mission statement.

Outline Expected Team Behaviors

Paint a clear picture of expected team behaviors. What broad behaviors are expected of people working together in teams? Include factors such as preferred conflict resolution process, decision-making tools, comfort with the acceleration or slowness of change, role model for new behaviors, and respect for the contributions of others. Include the accountability contract found in Chapter 4.

Identify New Workforce Competencies

Use expectations to define a set of new organizational competencies and skills-not position descriptions. What do you expect of the workforce for a team-based system to be successful? New behaviors can be technical (defined levels of computer literacy), team (positive group dynamics), or positional (manager as coach or CEO as system integrator).

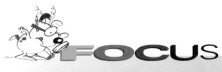

FOCUS

Preparing for Success

- Determine self-assessment methods.
- Conduct workforce self-assessment.
- Use a 360-degree process.
- Conduct competency development discussions.
- Plan training.
- Reevaluate competency achievement.

Assess and Prepare the Workforce for Team Success Factors

Identify tools for assessing level of competency development present in the organization. Ask every employee to participate in a self-assessment against the set of new organizational competencies. Use a 360-degree feedback process to maximize the quality of information. Conduct competency development discussions-individual, organizational focus groups, and teams. Create and implement a plan to develop and sustain new competencies, such as formal training, preceptor/mentor programs, team academy, or train the trainer. Recognize the critical nature of the training investment. Evaluate the acquisition of new competencies.

Carefully Prescribe the Handoff Process*

Significant ambiguity is associated with the transition of new functions to teams. People struggle with questions about who is supposed to do what and when they are supposed to be doing it. Without a clear handoff process, new team members may become easily overwhelmed and then resentful about "doing management's work." On the other hand, managers may feel anger and resentment about losing control over certain decisions to the team. Everyone must be held accountable to a clear set of guidelines governing just how and when to hand off new functions and decision making.

In a team-based system, teams take on functions traditionally performed by managers. If there is mass confusion about authority for decisions, management credibility and team performance will suffer.

Do the basics first, to minimize this confusion and resistance. Ask hard questions. Think through the process. What duties are now being performed by managers and staff groups? How will this change with the implementation of teams? Sort the tasks into categories aligned with the accountabilities now assigned to teams through the team charter, bylaws, or council accountabilities, based on the ultimate sharing of accountability

*Holpp L: If empowerment is good, why does it hurt? *Training* 32(3):52-58, 1995.

once the team-based system is fully operational. Organize the tasks into distinct categories (Orsburn et al., 1990):

1. Should be done by any team member
2. Should be performed by team leaders
3. Should be performed by management advisors to teams
4. Should be done by policy, procedure, or protocol
5. Should not be performed by teams
6. Should remain with management

See the Tool Chest at the end of this chapter for a handoff process. Be sure to determine what additional resources, tools, or protocols teams will need to successfully perform the new function. Learn to do each new function flawlessly. Treat every new function as if were your last. Add new functions as the previous ones are mastered. Repeat *ad infinitum* (Brooks, 1995).

Communicate the Team Charter

The team charter cannot function as a road map for the organization to guide transformation efforts if it is not shared. Consider having several town hall or focus group meetings to discuss the implications of the charter and to answer questions. Be sure to include team leaders as facilitators of the discussions. Opportunities to articulate their work will translate into quicker assimilation of this important information. See the sample town hall questions at the end of this chapter.

BEWARE OF THE DARK SIDE OF TEAM MENTAL MODELS

You must take considerable care in the chartering of teams, because the mental models you create can be flawed. The application of erroneous mental models will almost certainly produce team performance problems (Box 9-1).

Inaccuracies in mental models can lead team members to ignore discrepant information and perpetuate confusion. Team mental models can

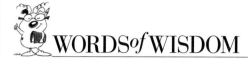

WORDS*of*WISDOM

It is no joke—leaders must be able to be taken seriously.

BOX **9-1**

Team Performance Problems and Poor Team Charters
• Inaccurate definitions of work and poor problem definitions
• Overreliance on shared information
• Negation of individual expertise in favor of shared vision
• False belief that everyone has to believe the same thing to come to consensus

BOX **9-2**

> ### *Example from the Field*
>
> A team became bogged down over the nature of its work to stimulate interest in clinical research. A strategic goal for this academic medical center was to demonstrate the effectiveness of the research being conducted in the organization. By the development and testing of new clinical practices, the organization hoped to establish its superiority in provide cutting edge care.
>
> A dominant subgroup in the newly formed team was composed of people who were researchers. Their specialty niche in the organization was to perform the research review process and participate in the conduct of research. By refusing to abandon this niche, they successfully influenced the team's work to support the conduct of nursing research. This was a flawed interpretation, because the expected outcome for this team was the development of new clinical practice protocols, derived from research, that would become a part of standard practice. Imagine their surprise when the team was disbanded because of inadequate organizational support and lack of funding!

Team concepts, expectations of relationships, values, beliefs, and ideologies are the stuff of team mental models.

also be significantly influenced by group dynamics early in the team experience. A subgroup can form to create a dominant view of the world. Other team members may struggle with this view, but if the subgroup is strong enough it can cause remaining team members to abandon the incorrect viewpoint and replace it with an incorrect but group-validated perspective. This dynamic is known as groupthink. Box 9-2 gives an example of team mental models.

ACKNOWLEDGE SOCIAL AND GROUP DYNAMIC FACTORS

In the public examination of one's knowledge as compared with another, important social forces are set into play. As I test my thoughts against yours in the chartering process, we challenge our individual self-concepts, risk taking, and commitment. It is important for management to acknowledge that these social and group dynamic factors are powerful variables that must be managed in health care settings. Teams are often made up of members from various functional departments, and members may hold various levels of positional authority in the organizational structure. It is no easy task for staff members to challenge managers or for managers to challenge their own boss, even in discussions of the team charter! As managers facilitate movement through the chartering methodology, be sure that group dynamics do not unintentionally create barriers to team performance. The challenge is to maintain balance between unity and diversity, creating enough commonality to maintain coordination but enough diversity to maximize coverage of all functions (Klimoski and Mohammed, 1994).

The personal dynamics of transformation to teams includes shifts in reality perception, one's role in the environment, and one's view of self. People construct their own perceptions about what the real organization is and is not. This information is used to identify individual beliefs about the essential functions of their work and their own personal definitions of their work. All members of the organization will need assistance in this developmental process:

1. *Anticipation:* A certain way of looking at self and others at work is challenged. This results in alterations in value and belief structures.
2. *Testing:* New beliefs about expected work behaviors are tested verbally or in action.
3. *Encounter:* Testing results in a feedback interaction.
4. *Confirmation/disconfirmation:* Alignment or discrepancy between real and perceived new behaviors occurs. This can be quite a surprise!
5. *Revision:* Feedback is accepted or rejected. Concept of self at work is adjusted.

The first year of implementation is critical in shaping people's new career identity, within the context of teams. Motivation, sense of competence, and personal definitions of success are influenced by the process used to manage change. The goal is to ensure that these personal factors are aligned with the beliefs, values, and expected behaviors of team-based systems.

THE ENERGIZING PERFORMANCE EFFECTS OF TEAM CHARTERS

Effective teams have energized and committed members who apply successful strategies in the development of work products to achieve organizational goals. This state of affairs occurs as team members, through experience, repeatedly apply their charter. Team charters are tools that can be applied by managers in examining the level of development of a team or the identification of barriers to performance.

Through a facilitated dialogue, all of the elements of the team charter are examined and reaffirmed. Chances are great that poorly performing teams or novice teams will not have fully developed shared visions.

The behavior over time (BOT) tool (see sample BOT tool at the end of this chapter) is a useful exercise to apply in this assessment (Anderson and Johnson, 1997).

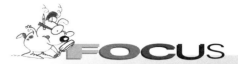

FOCUS

*The Process of Change in Self-Definition in Reorganized Workplaces**

1. Anticipation
2. Testing
3. Encounter
4. Confirmation/disconfirmation
5. Revision

*Fournier V, Payne R: Changes in self-construction during the transition from university to employment: a personal construct psychology approach, Journal of Occupational and Organizational Psychology 67(4):297-305, 1994.

ANTECEDENTS AND CONSEQUENCES OF TEAM CHARTERING METHODOLOGY

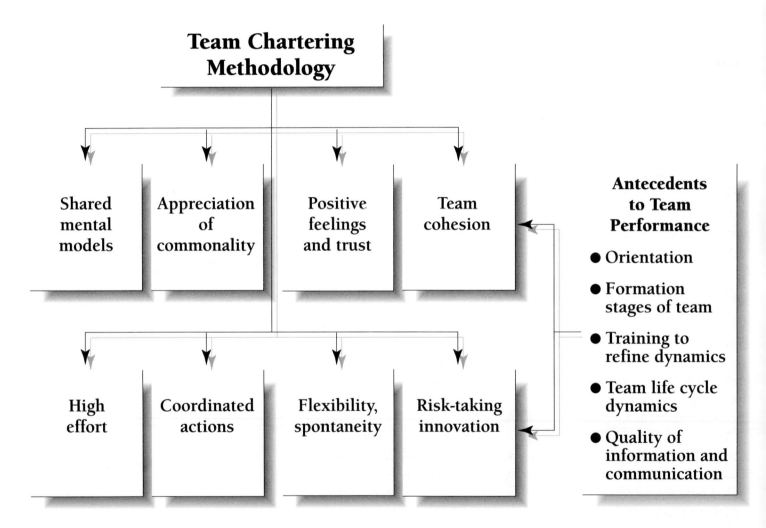

Clearly, the chartering methodology creates a team mental model that in turn affects team performance. How this process actually unfolds is depicted in the accompanying illustration.

As team members participate in the chartering process and then apply team norms in their work, shared mental models about the team are formed and imbedded as fact. The existence of shared mental models stirs feelings of connection and commonality within individual team members, and these feelings form the basis for trust and cohesion. At the team performance level, high effort, coordinated actions, flexibility, spontaneity, risk taking, and innovation are evident because of the presence of these individual personal and social factors.

OUTSIDE INFLUENCES ON TEAMS

What are the methods used to recruit and select team members, including the self-selection of leaders? Do members have the capacity for teamwork? A volunteer may have the commitment but lacks prerequisite skills. The process of membership selection is an emotional one. If not handled well, it can create considerable damage.

What prerequisite skills do team members need to bring with them? Training cannot provide all aspects of development for team members. It will not solve problems caused by a lack of personal insight, difficulty with authority, lack of clinical competence, or hidden agendas.

You must have a process for removing ineffective team members. How will people be removed in a manner that preserves self-esteem? Box 9-3 provides an example from the field.

The availability of training will provide opportunities for the refinement of team processes and expectations of competence. Life cycle dynamics of the team itself will influence success because of issues such as turnover vs. stagnant membership or establishing the right resource and communication networks.

BOX **9-3**

Example from the Field

In the early stage of a team's development a team leader had to be removed because of poor leadership skills, personal problems, or an unwillingness to share. How this individual was assisted in this transition forever influenced team norms. Communication errors and broken confidentiality agreements created a significant trust issue within the team. This was not identified by leaders, which resulted in mediocre team performance.

Beware of teams with long-term membership. They can cease to be effective because they talk only to each other or to outdated communication links (Klimoski, Mohammed, 1994). This is particularly true with health care teams that are assigned highly specialized functions.

Consider the impact of communication quality on the content of information within and outside the team. What is the predominant content of communications? Is there a form of team shorthand that describes team activities? Is it well understood? How is communication framed? Are problems seen as opportunities or threats? Are members "representing" their departments or arriving at the best decision for the patient? The language used by teams indicates predominant styles of influence, degree of openness to the rest of the organization, and willingness to negotiate position.

ALL STRESSED OUT AND NOWHERE TO GO

There is enduring preoccupation in health care organizations with leadership, as well as with the ambivalence with which it is viewed. The yearning for decisive leaders and the apprehension that they might upset the balance between power and autonomy has made us more adept at demanding leadership than truly embracing it.

Vigilance is the order of the day, in coaching, communicating, applying training, and reinforcing the team charter. In addition, the manager will model the belief that authority and accountability are shared by management and staff. If these activities are inadequate, the stress from trying to make an unsupported transformation work will stress people out.

A carefully crafted communication plan, drawn from the team charter, will assist you in the advisement of desired outcomes to teams. If it is clear and concise, this intercommunication will motivate teams to consistently evaluate their work in relationship to desired outcomes. It will also assist in the reinforcement of desired competencies.

Know when to train, when to sit on the sidelines, and when to assist people to leave their positions. Formal training is not always the answer. At the same time, if you are too quick to intervene, the team loses a precious opportunity to learn. Remember to be patient with both people and process.

Designing team-based systems and facilitating their implementation requires specific actions from managers.

Encourage teams to periodically ask several self-reflective questions:
- Where are we headed now?
- Are we on course?
- What is our team's unique role in this organization?
- What do we do well and what do we need to do better?
- How will the work of this team help us deliver better care?
- How will teams boost productivity and morale at the same time?
- Are we asking for and getting the resources that we need?
- Where do managers need to release control?
- Are we exercising the appropriate authority?

WORK SELF-CONCEPTS AND EFFECTIVE TEAMS

Most people have constructed through their formal education and work experience a self-concept that is unique to their workplace. In newly reorganized workplaces, this self-concept is shaken for just about everyone. No one feels like they "fit in" anymore, until the transformation is complete. Most people make the transition to a new self-concept. Those who cannot or will not make changes to their personal concept of work can wreak havoc in team-based systems:

- Teams spend an unnecessary amount of time trying to "convince" a team member about why a particular action is appropriate.
- Implementation plans are halted because management expresses a lack of confidence in teams.
- Hysteria erupts when a team makes a mistake.
- Continual questioning of decision-making authority wears everyone out.
- Blame for mediocre performance of teams or individuals reaches epidemic proportions.

The movement to a team-based organization is not a quick fix for financial or operational woes. It is not simply a nice thing to do for the staff. It is not a way to avert unionization. The transformation to a team-based system is a long-term commitment and a complex developmental transformation. All too often this fact is underestimated or undervalued.

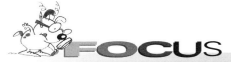

FOCUS

Dimensions of a Work Self-Concept

- Orientation toward people and moral themes
- Respect and fairness
- Work ethic
- Social aggression
- Task vs. people
- Achievement orientation
- Drive
- Priority of work
- Goal attainment methods
- Competence
- Efficiency
- New skills
- Confidence
- Relationships
- Abilities: self and others

THE TEAM CHARTER WORKSHOP

Instructions to Facilitator

1. Plan an informal social session to assist people in getting to know one another before the chartering session. Conduct a team-building exercise particularly if you are dealing with novice teams.

2. Allow at least 6 to 8 hours for the chartering workshop. One skilled facilitator can handle five teams.

3. Distribute the organization's mission statement, strategic plan, and any other materials you feel need to be referenced in the team charter. Do this at least 1 week before the chartering session. Attach the team charter preparation handout to the materials, which encourages participants to read and think about the information ahead of time.

4. Prepare a 10-minute "lecturette," defining for members why and how a team charter can enhance their performance.

5. Distribute the team charter worksheet. Review contents and time parameters.

6. Distribute a list of definitions so that there is a common starting place. For example, how does your organization define "customer"? "Patient care"?

7. Provide structure by limiting the time spent on each step of the chartering process.

8. Each team will need a flip chart to visually record its progress on each part of the charter. As each section is completed, have the team tape the flip chart paper for the section up on a wall before proceeding to the next step.

9. Large group sharing: allow the last hour of the day for each team to share its work product.

Bibliography

Anderson V, Johnson L: Four steps to graphing behavior over time, *The Systems Thinker* 8(3):8, 1997.

Brooks SJ: Managing a horizontal revolution, *Human Resources* 40(10):52-59, 1995.

Emery M: Mission control, *Training and Development* 50(7):51-54, 1996.

Fournier V, Payne R: Changes in self-construction during the transition from university to employment: a personal construct psychology approach, *Journal of Occupational and Organizational Psychology* 67(4):297-305, 1994.

Holpp L: If empowerment is good, why does it hurt? *Training* 32(3):52-58, 1995.

Klimoski R, Mohammed S: Team mental models: construct or metaphor? *Journal of Management* 20(2):403-438, 1994.

Orsburn JD et al: *Self-directed work teams,* Homewood, Ill, Business One Irwin, 1990.

Taincez G: Team playing: cross functional engineering teams, *Industry Week* 45(14):28-32, 1996.

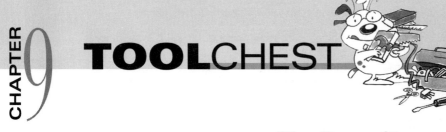

TOOLCHEST

CHAPTER 9

TOOLA: **The Team Charter Workshop**

Preparation Handout

Instructions: Please read and review the materials enclosed in your team charter workshop packet. You should have several documents that address the core values and strategic plan. To participate effectively in the workshop, please bring this completed worksheet with you. If you have any questions, do not hesitate to call

1. Have you ever seen any of the material in this packet before? (Circle One)   Yes   No

    If the answer was yes, how did your receipt of this information influence your work performance?

2. Do certain skills and behaviors expected of staff and managers stand out for you as you review each of the documents enclosed in this packet? If so, list them below:

3. What behaviors might these documents suggest you should expect of your colleagues?

4. What evidence should be used to judge whether you or your colleagues are performing in a manner suggested in these documents?

5. How might your team meet the performance requirements implied or stated in these documents?

6. Please jot down any other thoughts you have about what you read.

Team Charter Worksheet

Step 1: Team Mission Statement
- Try to limit the statement to no more than 10 sentences that address both the team's external and internal focus.
- Describe the team's external focus. Who are the team's customers? What are the team's critical network relationships? What does the team do for its customers?
- Describe the team's internal focus. What are the team's core values? What unique talents are represented on the team?

Step 2: Roles and Definitions
- Document the unique accountabilities for each team member: team leader, specialized role functions (such as information specialists, business advisors, finance), management coaches, and general expectations of every team member.
- Describe where the team fits in the organizational structure, team authority, place in the communication system, adjustments to the communication flow, feedback loops, and expected organizational outcomes.

Step 3: Team-Based System and the Strategic Plan
- Why do you believe teams will get you where you want to be?

- What will teams add to the accomplishment of the strategic plan for your organization?

Step 4: Expected Team Behaviors
- What do team members expect of each other?
- Include your team's accountability contract here.

Step 5: Workforce Competencies
- What changes do you expect in the work of your colleagues?
- List technical, team, and positional behaviors in competency terms.

Step 6: Prepare Workforce for Team Success

Describe how you will assist your colleagues in their self-assessment of new competencies.
- Consider a 360-degree feedback process to maximize understanding.
- How will you conduct competency discussions for individuals? For teams?
- How will you train people in the new behaviors?
- How will you evaluate the training and monitor organizational development?

Step 7: How Will New Functions Be Given to Teams?

- Carefully describe just what functions from what roles and positions will be transferred to teams.
- Prioritize this list and document how the handoff process will occur.

Step 8: Communicate the Team Charter

- How will you facilitate organizational members' knowledge of how to relate to teams?
- How will you help them understand where teams fit in the organizational structure, as well as the outcomes they can expect from teams?

Communicating the Team Charter

Sample Dialogue Questions for Town Hall Meetings

1. What are the hopes and dreams of staff members committed to team-based organizations?
2. What can working in teams contribute to a health care organization?
3. How does working in teams contribute to professional growth?
4. How can teams be implemented when we are in the middle of so much change?
5. Why would people resist working in teams?
6. How does organizing in teams relate to the work that we have already done?

Project Team Charter
John Doe Medical Center
Team Roles and Accountabilities
PROJECT CHAIR AND CO-CHAIR

Accountabilities: Project leaders are accountable for redesign success and provide daily project management.

Project leaders:
- Inspire people to action
- Maintain project balance between vision and practical realities
- Use awareness of organizational policies to build relationships and commitment
- Communicate and negotiate among diverse groups of special interests
- Sell policy changes
- Assist project team in acquiring and maintaining power and credibility
- Are action oriented but delegate
- Make sure project remains a high priority in the organization
- Link and coordinate the work of the project team
- Ensure a disciplined process of redesign is applied by the project team

Project Team Charter
John Doe Medical Center
THE EXECUTIVE COACHES—ORIGINAL ACTION
  SPONSORS

Accountabilities: Act as organizational sponsors who acquire the necessary resources to the project team, including access to information and people.

Executive Coaches:

- Acquire and maintain funding and long-term support for implementation
- Speak to reluctant peers and subordinates to facilitate their involvement in the project
- Assist project team and work groups in overcoming organizational obstacles to change, including departmental, political, and cultural barriers
- Attend project team meetings
- Speak at organizational meetings where project is being discussed
- "Walk the talk" by participating in education or awareness building activities (in person or on video).
- Make necessary policy changes so that patient/family centered care can be successfully implemented
- Communicate upward to CEO, chief of medical staff, and board to ensure organization-wide support.
- Clear calendars of participants to ensure involvement on project teams and work groups
- Assist executive team members in incorporating implementation goals in each of their direct reports and performance plans, and hold them accountable
- Update project team in external events and situations that may influence implementation

Project Team Charter
John Doe Medical Center
SPECIFIC PROJECT TEAM ROLES

Accountabilities: To provide expert support to the work of the project team.

1. *Business specialist:*
   - Incorporates the operational implications in project team's decision making
   - Holds managerial position
   - Ensures that operational issues arise in redesign planning and implementation
2. *Information specialist:*
   - Communicates multilayered description of information systems technology to a variety of diverse users
   - Explains technological options and risks to project teams
   - Assists work team in the design of IS technology contemplated for redesign
   - Suggests alternatives for technology support
   - Leads IS departments shift in vision and activity to patient/family centered approach
3. *Financial specialist:*
   - Assists project directors and project team in the analysis of financial data
   - Facilitates creation of financial data for purposes of project evaluation and tracking costs against budget
   - Assists project units in realignment of financial reporting and budgeting that reflects new patient/family centered delivery system
4. *Knowledge coordinator:*
   - Is fluent with PCs and project management software
   - Maintains project information outcomes tracking, project documentation and redesign tools, distribution lists, meeting minutes, project history files, presentations, correspondence, and workshops (equipment and tools)

TOOL B: Analyzing Team Performance Over Time[*]

Instructions: This tool helps you see beyond the emotion of the moment and identify patterns of team behavior that are not aligned with the charter or may be dysfunctional in nature. Called a behavior-over-time graph (Anderson and Johnson, 1997), it is *not* meant to be used as a quantification instrument. Do not expect to record precise values. The exercise is designed for you to see how a problem's parts are connected. Then you can take steps to determine where the greatest opportunity for intervention may be located.

Step 1: Team Dialogue: Describe What Is Happening

Using the questions found on page XXX, have team members discuss where they see their team's performance at this moment in time. For example: "We are meeting more often but we are still behind on our time lines." "People are delegating more but the work is not getting done." "We are making decisions, but some of them are not being supported by management."

Step 2. Create Focusing Questions

With your team, decide on focus questions that get to the heart of the problem. Do not mince words or try to make the questions safe.
- How come, if we are doing the right work, we are not producing the right outcomes?
- Why aren't we using the tools/technology we learned in the course of performing the team's work?

Step 3: Identify Key Variables

Using a brainstorming process, identify the critical variables that your team thinks may be related to the problem, such as incomplete handoff process, layoff action and change in team membership, mistake made by team, or management distrust of teams.

[*] Anderson V, Johnson L: Four steps to graphing behavior over time, *The Systems Thinker* 8(3):8, 1997.

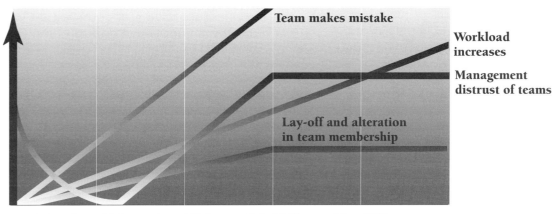

Jun 1996	Sep 1996	Dec 1996	Feb 1997	May 1997	

Step 4: Sketch a Graph

After drawing your graph, use it to discuss the interrelationships of factors influencing team development or performance. How did the layoff affect the team and its work processes? How was decision making impaired? How did the changes in everyone's workload affect team processes and management faith in teams?

TOOL C: The Handoff Plan

Instructions: Team members must have already been selected and have participated in the team chartering workshop. Managers and team members sit down together to plan the handoff process, using the team charter as a guide. A facilitator conducts the planning session.

Step 1: Identifying the What

Review management job descriptions and the team charter. If you need more information, consider having managers keep an activity log for 1 week and bring those logs to the planning session.

Step 2: Identifying the Who

Group all of the management activities into the following categories:
The team should take on now:
• The team leader or management advisor to the team should assume this now.
• This task needs to be returned to another department.

• The team should take on eventually:
• This task needs to be put into policy and procedure.
• We all need to stop doing this task.

Step 3: Identify the How

Describe the processes needed to accompany the shift in accountability. Include policies and procedures, process descriptions, and forms that accompany performance of the function. It is also helpful to flow chart the "before and after" picture.

Step 4: Identify the When

Apply project management tools to create a time line with accountabilities for the handoff process. You should have a document that lists the time for the transition. Leave enough time for the transition process.

10

Good Team Outcomes: The Promise and the Reality

THE PROMISE OF TEAM-BASED ORGANIZATIONS

In a team-based system, a guiding principle is the recognition of the interconnectedness of everyone to everything. This principle demands that the congealed patterns of fragmentation, competition, and reactivity be dissolved in an organization. Instead, new opportunities are taken to connect teamwork, apply creative solutions, and to use intuition (Wilson, 1994). The diversity within cross-functional health care teams creates a new culture of leadership. It is the context in which team outcomes are achieved. In effective teams, there is continual acknowledgment of each other's contributions to the delivery of care, real authority to make changes, and control over health care practices. The freedom to apply these valuable human resources is accompanied by accountability for either actions taken or failure to act (Box 10-1).

- Patient care improves with teams, in the form of value-added service, shorter time to implementation, and quicker application of new knowledge.
- Certain organizational benefits, including greater productivity, more effective use of resources, better problem solving, innovation, and higher-quality decisions, can be expected from team-based systems.

BOX 10-1

Superior Teams

- Maximize use of team resources
- Superior output against all odds
- Leadership focused on teamwork

Team member feelings:
- Inclusion
- Commitment
- Loyalty
- Pride
- Trust

- Most organizations report a 20% to 40% gain in productivity resulting from deep employee involvement (Orsburn et al, 1990).
- Benefits to team members have included authority to do what is right or needed. More personal pride in the quality of services, a feeling of ownership, enhanced collegiality, development of personal leadership, and challenge have been gains for organizational members participating in teams.

THE REALITY OF TEAM-BASED ORGANIZATIONS

Unfortunately, team-based systems fail in many health care organizations. Why? One explanation is that the organization's cultural fabric is significantly challenged, with a new model of empowerment and leadership at the point of service. Team life in health care organizations is difficult because of rivalry, authority, dependency, and leadership issues. Two characteristics of health care cultures limit the success of teams: the use of collegiality to avoid the politics of group life and the dependent nature of organizational relationships.

Collegiality: Blessing or Curse?

Many people involved in the delivery of health care have been taught to act as colleagues. At face value this seems to be a good thing, but collegiality can also be used to avoid the true work of teams. Why does this happen?

Professional socialization teaches people to resist team life, because the emphasis in formal and informal training is on individual rather than group performance. Reward systems at work are similar, recognizing only individual achievement.

Health care workers fear that teams will limit their professional authority, prevent them from exercising their best judgments, dictate what they are to do next, or replace them with less-educated providers. These fears are based on the false belief that if people succumb to working in a team, they will somehow constrain each other through the team's actions.

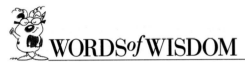

WORDS*of*WISDOM

Teams are not ends unto themselves . . . they are a means to achieve other organizational goals.

Consequently, team members are nice to each other, most often when they disagree the most. Under the guise of collegiality, decisions are diluted so as to please everyone and thus have minimum impact. Real differences are avoided for fear of retribution. There is fear about being controlled and, at the same time, a wish to be led by powerful others. People mistakenly believe that they are acting collaboratively and are surprised when they learn differently.

A culture of dysfunctional collegiality is marked by split views of leaders (tyrants or patrons), reward systems that do not acknowledge real differences in performance, teams made up of the weakest people, and an overall sense of drift or uncertainty (Hirschlorn, 1989).

Dependence: Our Health Care Legacy

The implementation of team-based systems is made more difficult by the dependent nature of health care organizational culture. What does a culture of dependency look like?

- A cultural context of dependence on rules and "following orders" instead of thinking for oneself.
- Ambivalence between a wish for a democratic culture and demands for all-powerful leaders.
- Aggression is the antithesis of caring and must be inhibited.
- Always meeting the needs of others. Standing apart, blowing your own horn, and self-promotion are not permissible.

Box 10-2 provides an example from the field. What happened in this example? The reward system in this culture put the burden on those people most strongly committed to patient care, while the rest of the people were uncorrected for failure to participate in problem solving. Committed individuals soon found themselves overburdened. Organizational members overrelied on these people. When they attempted to resolve the staffing problem, they were treated poorly. Such experiences can strike fear and inconsistency in leaders, who then in turn develop an intolerance for mistakes and a strong tendency to blame (Hirsahborn, 1989).

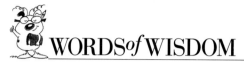

WORDS of WISDOM

As William Faulkner once observed: the past is never dead and buried . . . in fact it is not even past!

~

If teams are to deliver on their promise, the mutuality of collegial relationships must be enacted as a strength instead of a defense against the politics of organizational life.

BOX **10-2**

Example from the Field: "Good Nurses"

A team of health care professionals was always willing to work extra hours, even though they were exhausted. They were openly recognized as "good staff," but privately described as being "only out for themselves." Staffing problems had been an issue for at least 6 months. Initially, the team led an attempt to resolve inequities in staffing resources across the patient care division. When all of the team leaders in the division came together in an attempt to resolve the problem, real differences dissipated the cloak of collegiality. Members attacked each other's ideas and then turned on the people who had requested the meeting. There was no interpersonal system for genuine problem solving. Leadership was devalued and real differences were unresolved. The staffing problem continued, and the committed work team had several resignations, including its leader.

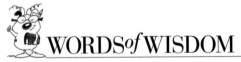

WORDS*of*WISDOM

External control may correct errors . . . but only internal relationships can prevent their occurrence!

Leaders and committed individuals cannot sustain their efforts forever. When this happens, the organization is left without a way to move forward with goal achievement. New leaders replace old ones in a revolving door. Soon no one wants a leadership role.

Cultural characteristics can inhibit teams from addressing the good and the bad in their relationships and prevent the development of the strong interpersonal systems necessary to team success.

BUILDING CULTURAL INTERVENTIONS

The cultural context of health care organizations can impede the effectiveness of a team-based system, through the reinforcement of several kinds of dysfunctional organizational behaviors. For example, holding on to the view that "we are all one big family" can preclude leaders from taking action to remove incompetent but senior "family members"! The culture simply supports substandard performance.

When teams are implemented in a culture that fiercely maintains collegiality and devalues independence, real issues rarely surface. Passion about anything is limited, so as to protect people's vulnerability. Caution in action is the watchword. Outcome achievement is diminished.

Leaders must assist team members to understand that the capacity for successful outcomes means that members respect each other's contributions and can trust one another to be honest. In effective teams, members do not feel pressured to always have the "right" answer. They can depend on one another to use their skill and knowledge effectively.

The decline of many team-based systems can be linked to adhering to a strong culture that was appropriate in the past but is now out of sync with the team environment. Be sure to conduct an honest cultural assessment before the implementation of a team-based system. This process will assist organizational members in identifying those aspects of the health care culture that could limit team success. Through focus group discus-

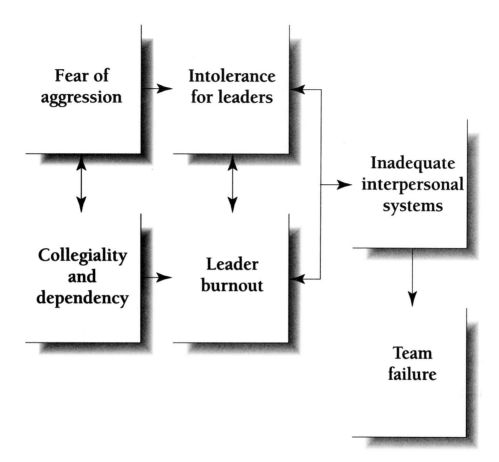

sions, team meetings, or interviews, people can identify the degree of fit between a team-based approach and the current culture. When the features of an organization's culture are well understood, reward systems can be fashioned that fit the desired culture. (See Cultural Assessment Tool at the end of this chapter.)

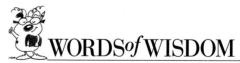

WORDS*of*WISDOM

The greatest challenge in team-based systems is finding champions willing to pursue the vision and deal with the ramifications of politics and culture.

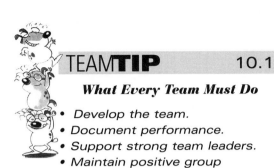

TEAMTIP   10.1

What Every Team Must Do

- *Develop the team.*
- *Document performance.*
- *Support strong team leaders.*
- *Maintain positive group dynamics.*
- *Reward team outcomes.*

CYCLE 1
Team
structuring

CYCLE 3
Team
organization

CYCLE 2
Team development

TRAP-PROOFING YOUR TEAMS

To develop teams in such a way that they produce value-added outcomes is a major challenge. From the time a team is chartered, there must be purposeful actions to avoid the team traps of failure to invest in team development, inadequate performance measurement, deficient team leadership, and dysfunctional team dynamics (Team Tip 10-1).

TEAM DEVELOPMENT

Team leaders have an enormous accountability for understanding and facilitating team development. All teams move through three developmental cycles. Each demands a different performance from leaders, and each has its own distinct set of predictable outcomes (Greene, 1995).

Cycle 1

Team structuring occurs early in a team's life. This cycle entails all of the behaviors team members enact to define their collective relationships as a team. People are challenged to understand what it means to be a member of a work team. They are not just a group of passive workers asked to give "input" but a team assigned serious organizational accountabilities, with high expectations for performance.

People reveal many ways of integrating personal definitions of work with expectations for team success. Some members may silently watch the leader in an attempt to identify which behaviors are acceptable. Others form alliances with subgroups. These may or may not be helpful. Still others test the water and assert themselves. As the team progresses through this team infrastructure cycle, people become more secure as they discover what they are supposed to do and start doing it. Team structuring is an intense experiential learning cycle that produces clarity of team purpose and work processes.

Team member behaviors include the following:
- Testing each other and articulating definitions of the team's work
- Identifying which people have influence and control

- Asking for suggestions and feedback
- Establishing ground rules via accountability contracts
- Settling on work methods
- Identifying opportunities for shared leadership vs. individual leadership
- Testing to see how much of the team issues the leader will own.

Team leader goals this cycle include the following:

- Equalize participation levels
- Reinforce accountability contract and team norms
- Modify individual behaviors to team behaviors without inhibiting individual effort
- Apply team performance measures to evaluate accountability
- Delineate contracts, equity of participation, and definitions of teamwork and commitment

Cycle 2

Team development is the second cycle. Leadership is established and rules of conduct formalized. The team develops and tests a variety of work processes. Some will be incorporated into formal team processes and some will fail miserably. Important outcomes of this cycle are the identification and application of effective team systems in the process of outcome achievement.

Team member behaviors include the following:

- Immersion in the work of the team
- Increased confidence in team charter
- Strong team orientation
- Unconditional regard for each other
- Resistance to the addition of new members or change in leadership
- Practicing new methods of problem solving and goals achievement

Team leader goals this cycle include the following:

- Develop strong decision-making, conflict-resolution, consensus-building, and feedback methods.

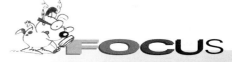

Elements of a Developed Team

- People choose to be on the team.
- People own their actions.
- There is a stated commitment to the team.
- There is room for both individual and team goals.
- Communication is action oriented:
To the person who is able to act
To move the team forward
- Formal processes exist for accomplishing the team's work.

- Monitor and intervene in dependent team relationships or dysfunctional collegiality.
- Document outcomes.
- Apply performance measures.

Cycle 3

Team optimization is that cluster of activities which clearly reflect that the team is well developed and able to effectively contribute to organizational goals. It can take up to 5 years to create optimized teams! The outcomes of this cycle are formal acceptance of teams as the "norm" for the organization, continuous improvement, and value-added outcomes.

Team member behaviors include the following:

- Team risk taking and significant challenges to the organization's status quo
- Actual outcome achievement
- Momentum and excitement about the team's contributions to organizational goals
- Pride in team membership
- Clarity in understanding what it means to work as a team as opposed to ways of working in the past
- Coaching new teams

Team leader goals this cycle include the following:

- Sustaining team ownership of process, product, and outcomes
- Application of performance measures to document real outcomes
- Communication of team outcomes to stakeholders
- Continuous learning
- Balancing dialogue, advocacy, and inquiry in team interactions (Convey, 1994)

Interactions among team members while engaged in work are most effective when they are characterized by dialogue, advocacy, and inquiry. The team leader's job is to ensure that no one pattern of interaction dominates the work processes employed by the team. Dialogue is the capacity to listen carefully to another person's point of view to fully understand that person. This is different from mentally preparing a response. Advocacy is the practice of persuasion and influencing the team to take a particular position. Inquiry is asking thoughtful and critical questions in exploring an issue. Effective team communications balance these interactions. Ineffective teams allow members to delay or obstruct decision making by overreliance on advocacy or inquiry. For example, team members who assume the ever popular "devil's advocate" role can stall team movement for quite some time!

PERFORMANCE MEASUREMENT

Team performance levels must be measured to maximize team performance. A multitude of instruments are available to team leaders interested in developing a compendium of performance measurement tools (see Tool Chest). Each method contributes in its own unique way to the facilitation of effective teams.

Information collected from team performance measures can be used to do the following:
- Document how crucial the work of the team is to the organization
- Validate accomplishments and team growth, which motivates and stimulates greater team momentum
- Identify cultural drivers and barriers to movement through the team development cycle
- Diagnose team problems and test effects of interventions
- Clarify strategies, tactics, or new directions for problem solving

Several issues must be considered before embarking on a team performance process. First, what kinds of teams will you be evaluating? Many people have difficulty describing just what kinds of team are operating in their organization. Remember, different teams have different structures, member composition, and accountabilities. Can you really compare the performance of a project team with a multidisciplinary patient care team? Differences must be acknowledged before measurement.

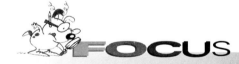

FOCUS

Team Player Competencies
- *Rational problem-solving skills*
- *Interpersonal skills:*
  Respect
  Mutuality
- *Value for learning*
- *Action orientation*
- *Strong volunteerism*
- *Self-direction*
- *Effective delegation*

Second, most health care employees have not been held accountable for team behaviors. Have you defined what it means to be a team player? (Your team charter should have helped you with this work.) What are the competencies that teams must demonstrate in their daily work?

Third, there are special considerations to be addressed when measuring the performance of cross-functional teams. Diversity in membership certainly facilitates comprehensive decision making and parallels the multidisciplinary nature of health care delivery. Because members will differ in educational preparation, life stage, and professional orientation, they will develop at different rates. Interpretation of team performance must take into consider that team members will vary significantly in their strengths and weaknesses.

Finally, in this age of health care report cards, recognize that some team performance measures will be attacked as "soft" and unmeasureable. One cannot "count" human behavior. Keep in mind that while quantification methods do document some team outcomes, qualitative performance measures help you to precisely describe why or why not you got where you needed to be (Greene, 1995).

Performance Measure Checklist

Teams struggle with documenting their performance. They may attempt to identify outcomes that are unrealistic for their stage of development. They may be unclear about what kinds of teams are being evaluated. This checklist will help teams determine the best approach to performance measurement by helping teams understand just what they are measuring and why.

Type of team

- What kind of team are you evaluating? A project team? A work team? A CQI team?
- What work products are expected from the kind of team you are evaluating?

Team player competencies

- What behaviors do you expect to see enacted by team members?
- What changes in workforce behaviors are you expecting as the result of this team's work?
- What is it like to work on this team?
- How similar or different are the members of this team? How does this affect our performance?

Team development

- What is our developmental stage?
- What outcomes should we expect from our work at this stage of our team's development?

Four Types of Performance Measures

Milestones

Milestones are points of demarcation in a process, representing the completion of a specific cluster of team activity producing an outcome at a certain point in time. They can boost team morale and inspire action, particularly during times of difficult transition. Milestone measurement must be sequenced well, with points far enough apart that achievements are clearly present or absent.

Rating systems

Rating systems are basically charts completed at the end of designated times, such as quarterly team evaluation sessions. They are also a part of workshops designed to strengthen team performance. The rating systems identify positive team characteristics that ensure potent team outcomes. Team members, a team observer, or an outside facilitator typically use such instruments to provide feedback on the efficiency of team work processes.

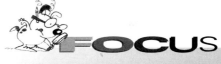

Team Performance Measures

- *Milestone*
- *Rating systems*
- *Peer review*
- *Self-assessment*

Peer review

Peer review occurs when team members evaluate each other's performance and provide feedback and recommendations. Typically these methods are found in the structure of reports by task force leaders or subgroups reporting to the team. The need to provide a structure for such reports is commonly overlooked, which diminishes the performance measurement value of this method. The focus of evaluation must be on the quality of the work performed, the comprehensiveness of the work, and the involvement of key stakeholders in recommendation development. (See *Peer Review: Task Force Recommendation to Team* at the end of this chapter.)

Self-assessment

Self-assessment methods are largely developmental tools. Their application facilitates evaluation of team dynamics. Their completion by team members provides opportunities for people to voice concerns about team competency, clarify the work, and select strategies for strengthening team operations. The developmental cycles of a team, tools appropriate to that cycle, and a list of performance measure tools found at the end of this chapter are summarized in Table 10-1.

When teams are properly led and properly monitored, they can make potent contributions to organizational goals and tackle major obstacles along the way.

TABLE 10-1

Performance Measurement Tools and Developmental Cycle

DEVELOPMENTAL CYCLE	PERFORMANCE MEASUREMENT METHOD	SAMPLE TOOLS
Team Building	• Self-assessments	• Building team commitment • What do we expect?
Team Development	• Behavioral exercises • Rating systems • Peer reviews	• Focusing on conflict • Task force report
Team Optimization	• Milestones • Peer review	• Implementation methodology

TEAM LEADERSHIP

The performance of the team leader is a critical factor in the success of teams. Much has been written about the team leader (Porter-O'Grady and Wilson, 1995). All the descriptions have one key theme in common: the leader ensures a balance between team task and process.

Team Leader as Task Master

Eliminates cross-functional barriers and excessive procedure

Patient centered

Outcomes driven

Technical skills: leadership (mission and values); project management; communication, facilitation, training, consulting, and problem solving

Team Leader as Interpersonal System Manager

Empowers the team

Teacher and counselor

Listeners not tellers

Open, honest, and worthy of trust

Establishes fair work processes

See mistakes as learning opportunities

TEAM DYNAMICS

A keystone to team effectiveness is the nature of team member interactions in relationship to their task and performance charter. While much has been written about team dynamics, some issues are particularly important to consider for health care teams: conflict management methods, understanding the principles of consensus decision making, and applying organizational discipline.

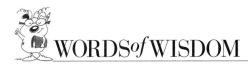

WORDS of WISDOM

When people's interests are involved and they are given influence and opportunity . . . they will commit to find the time to solve the problem!

What Kind of Conflict Does Your Team Have?

Conflict is a natural part of team process. It is what makes team decision making so effective in the first place! Effective teams know how to manage their conflict so that it produces a positive contribution. Less effective teams hide behind collegiality and ignore conflict altogether or allow it to produce outcomes that inhibit success. Two types of team conflict are common: C-type, or cognitive conflict; and A-type, or animosity-based conflict (Amason et al, 1995).

C-type conflicts, or cognitive disputes, improve team effectiveness

C-type conflicts arise when teams focus on issues of substance. Team members naturally bring different ideas, opinions, and perspectives to the table. This type of conflict requires teams to focus attention on unconscious assumptions underlying a particular issue. Conflict exposes such conjectures and fosters an exploration of alternative ideas.

C-type conflict fosters acceptance of the final decision by all of the team members because of enhanced understanding of other people's point of view. Frank discussions, integration of multiple perspectives, and the exploration of differences provides the foundation for team "buy-in" for the final decision.

A-type conflicts are animosity based and get in the way of success

A-type conflict undermines team effectiveness by blocking interpersonal effectiveness. The team climate is riddled with cynicism, distrust, and avoidance. The quality of decisions declines because commitment to the team is eroded. People are simply not willing to engage in the type of discussions necessary for successful team action.

People who are distrustful, hostile, or cynical are unlikely to support decisions made by the team. If a decision should be made, team members do not understand it or each other's point of view. They undermine implementation efforts and distance themselves from the team's decision. People

Steps in Managing Conflict

1. Stay focused on the main conflict.
2. Think outside the box.
3. Make communication safe.
4. Integrate everyone's knowledge.

who have experienced potent A-type conflict usually reduce their participation in future meetings or resign from the team.

How to manage "C" while not getting trapped in "A"*

- *Focused activity.* Stick closely to the task at hand. Do not allow sidetracking, hidden agendas or trivial disputes to delay resolution. Prepare for conflict. Teams comfortable with conflict get right to the point. (See *Four Tips for Managing Conflict in Work Teams* at end of this chapter.)
- *Think outside the box.* Think beyond the normal options. Teams possess the potential to integrate the strongest thoughts, knowledge, and experiences of their members.
- *Safe communication.* Speak freely and challenge viewpoints. Communication in teams should be free of censorship, anger, resentment, or retribution.
- *Integration.* Make the fullest use of team members. Avoid unequal participation because the end result may be the opinions of the strongest or most vocal members. Seek out the feedback of less verbal members and moderate those who are the most vocal.

Blame: A Conflict Generator

More than any other dynamic, blame has the power to stop a team in its tracks. Health care professionals are naturally error averse. This attitude is essential to matters of patient care but deadly in any other kind of work because there is no room for error. Whenever something goes wrong, there is always the search for a guilty party. Once that person or group has been discovered and labeled, the anxiety about the problem is diminished and the problem is believed to be solved. When it surfaces later, this conflict cycle repeats itself. Blame rarely enhances our understanding of the prob-

*Amason AC, Hochwater WA, Thompson KR, Harrison AN: Conflict: an important dimension to successful management teams, *Organizational Dynamics*, 24(2):20-36, 1995.

lem or creates new solutions. The opposite of blame is accountability. To be accountable means that the team or individual members can be counted on to keep agreements, accept responsibility, and perform their work to their best ability.

To avoid the tendency to blame, do the following (Paul, 1997):

- Define and assign responsibilities in advance.
- Conduct contracting discussions in groups, along with a commitment to avoid blame and focus on accountability.
- Remember that others are acting rationally from their own perspective. it may not be rational to you but it is to them.
- Realize that you probably have contributed in some way to the current problem.
- Remind yourself that judgment and criticism mask vision.

Consensus Decision Making

Consensus decision making is one of the most commonly misunderstood work processes. Many teams fail to reach consensus because they do not use formal ground rules or consensus tools. (See *Team Consensus Worksheet* at end of this chapter.) Yet ground rules help members develop a mental picture of the behaviors needed to reach consensus.

Consensus decision making ensures that each member's choice is a free one, to which he or she commits. The process of understanding every person's perspective equalizes the distribution of power and participation. Each member's concern must be heard; each member's support is necessary.

Ground Rules for Consensus Decision Making

1. *Test assumptions and inferences.* Do not assume something to be true unless you have verified it. Do not infer conclusions about things you do not know based on things you do know.
2. *Share all relevant information.* Both facts and feelings are relevant information. Articulate concerns in a manner that fosters understanding of your experience.

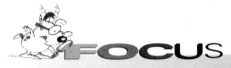

FOCUS

Consensus Decision Making: How Do You Know You Are There?

My personal views and ideas have been listened to and considered.

I have had the opportunity to listen and consider the views of every other team member in our discussion of this issue.

Even if this decision was not my choice, I can support it and work toward its implementation.

3. *Focus on interests, not positions or solutions.* At the beginning of the discussion, each team member should state his or her personal interest in the issue at hand. Why is it important? What do you hope to see accomplished here? Solutions can be conflicting even when interests are compatible.

4. *Be specific; use examples.* Describe the observable behaviors or outcomes that will result should the team adopt your position. Agree on the meaning of important words. "This is what this word means to me. Does it mean the same thing for you?"

5. *Explain the reasons behind statements, questions, and behavior.* Tell other people why you are doing what you are doing. "I am not participating in the discussion right now because I am reflecting on what Jenny just said." Or "When I am silent it does not mean that I agree or disagree." Help people interpret your behavior correctly.

6. *Disagree openly with team members.* Open disagreement tests inferences and assumptions. It the foundation of valid information. Unchallenged assumptions can lead to poor solutions.

7. *Test disagreements.* Design ways of testing disagreements. Apply CQI techniques such as value analysis to verify individual member predictions. Ask "Could both be correct?" (See *Team Consensus Worksheet* at end of this chapter.)

8. *Always discuss the undiscussables.* Team members sometimes need to open up forbidden topics to share valid information.

ORGANIZATIONAL DISCIPLINE

When discipline is absent from team efforts, solutions suffer from incomplete implementation because crucial steps are overlooked. Inadequate information, authority, resources, and influence plague the work of the team. Tough decisions are not made because they are unrecognized.

- In disciplined teams, there are clearly identified outcomes and indicators for any major task. These outcomes are negotiated and committed to by each and every team member. By clearly defining anticipated outcomes at the beginning, problems such as inadequate resources for implementation or lack of organizational support can be addressed in time to avoid failure.

- A clear team infrastructure is documented. There is a formal approach to chartering teams. A common set of team strategies is applied to work problems. Member roles and competencies are delineated.
- An implementation methodology is consistently applied. Team leaders are skilled in project management technology.

Team-based systems suffer from many traps that, if not ameliorated, can derail team efforts and spiral downward all evidence of team performance. Teams cannot recover from organizational blunders in their development. The collision of work cultures can have crippling effects, particularly if cultural strategies are poorly thought out and implemented in a careless or haphazard manner. If teams are not developed by leaders, early successes may be dismissed as flukes because there has been no transfer of learning. If performance problems are unidentified or misunderstood, there will be a strong decline in team performance. The key to successful team outcomes is to keep teams at the heart of all work performed, insist on leadership, and always focus on team capability.

Bibliography

Amason A, Hochwater WA, Thompson KR, Harrison AW: Conflict: an important dimension in successful management of teams, *Organizational Dynamics* 24(2):Autumn, 20-36, 1995.

Convey SC: Performance management in cross-functional teams, *CMA-The Management Accounting Magazine* 69(8): October, 13-16, 1994.

Greene RJ: Culturally compatible reward strategies, *ACA Journal* 40(3): Autumn, 60-71, 1995.

Hirschhorn L: Professionals, authority and group life: a case study of a law firm. In Hirschhorn L, Barrett C, eds: *The psychodynamics of organizations,* Philadelphia, Temple University Press, 1989.

Klimoski R, Mohammed S: Team mental models: construct or metaphor? *Journal of Management* 20(2):403–438, 1994.

Paul M: Moving from blame to accountability, *The Systems Thinker* 9(1)1-6: February 1997.

Porter O'Grady T, Wilson CK: *The leadership revolution in health care,* Gaithersburg, Md, Aspec Publications, 1995.

Orsburn JD, Moran J, Musselwhite E, Zenter JH: *Self-directed work teams,* Homewood, Ill, Business One Irwin, 1990.

Schwartz RM: Ground rules for groups, *Training and Development* 45(7): August, 45-52, 1994.

Senge P, Kleiner A, Roberts C, Ross R, Smith B: *The fifth discipline fieldbook,* New York, Doubleday.

Wilson CK: The new business paradigm: demands for nursing leadership, *Aspens Advisor for Nurse Executives* 9(8):3–6, 1994.

Wilson CK: Organizational discipline, *Aspen's Advisor for Nurse Executives* 10(11):2-3, August 1995.

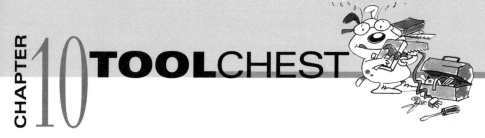

TOOL CHEST

TOOL A: Cultural Assessment Tool

Instructions: The periodic assessment of your culture is an investment in maintaining the effectiveness of a team-based system.

Objectives:

1. To examine the beliefs and values of key stakeholder groups in an organization before the implementation of a team-based system for monitoring congruence with team principles.
2. To determine gaps between stakeholder groups.
3. To create a forum for cultural dialogue.

Time requirement: 90 minutes per focus group

Supplies: cultural assessment questionnaires, a flip chart, and markers

Method:

1. Prepare a list of the key stakeholders to be included in this assessment. Consider not only those in formal stakeholder positions but also formal and informal subgroups.
2. Before eliciting input, explain to participants the mission and charter of the team-based system and how it relates to the organization's goals. Make clear the realities that the organization faces in the implementation of teams. (Structure your comments so that participants understand the cultural characteristics needed to support team success.)
3. Distribute the first copy of the cultural assessment questionnaire. Ask people to think about what the culture is at this point in time and then to complete the survey.
4. Distribute the second copy of the survey, which has been copied on a different color of paper. Now ask respondents to answer according to what they believe the culture should be, if teams are to be successful.
5. Put three headings across the top of the flip chart: *current culture, desired culture gap,* and *strategy.* List the question numbers on the left side of the flip chart. Work through each of the questions and record respondent conclusions.
6. Once everyone has provided their input, discuss the feedback. Use the following focus questions: Why does the gap exist? How critical is it to close each gap? What are the consequences of not closing each gap? How can we go about closing these gaps? How will we know if we are successful?

Cultural Assessment Tool

This assessment tool has been adapted for team-based systems from Greene.*

Instructions:

1. Please review each of the questions below. You will be given two copies of this questionnaire. On the first copy, circle the number closest to your beliefs about how our organization really works.
2. After you have finished, receive a second copy of the instrument. Now think about how our organization *needs* to operate, if our teams are to be successful.
3. Once you have completed the two forms, use the Gap Analysis Worksheet to identify differences between how we work now and how we need to work.

1. Performance is defined as:

1	2	3	4	5

- Budgets being met
- Individual action
- What the boss wants
- Patient needs met
- Team action
- What patients need

2. Good performance is because of:

1	2	3	4	5

- A few key people
- Individual determination
- Working within the rules
- Everyone
- Shared destiny
- Challenging assumptions

3. Success is defined in terms of:

1	2	3	4	5

- Job descriptions
- Organizational goals
- Short term
- Quick fix
- Competencies
- Team goals
- Long term
- Sustainability

4. Information is:

1	2	3	4	5

- Individual power
- Tightly managed
- What the boss wants
- Critical to teams
- Flowing in all directions
- What patients need

5. Management is:

1	2	3	4	5

- Layered
- Control
- Policy and procedure
- Flat
- Resource
- Values and vision

6. The future requires:

1	2	3	4	5

- Financial rigor
- Improved services
- Continuous improvement
- Financial investment
- New services
- Balanced risk

Greene RJ: Culturally compatible rewards strategies, *ACA Journal* 40(3):60-71, 1995.

7. People are managed as if they are:				
1	2	3	4	5

- Children
- Costs
- Task oriented

- Adults
- Assets
- Outcomes oriented

8. Resources are allocated:				
1	2	3	4	5

- To individuals
- To the winners
- From manager self-interest

- To support team performance
- To add value
- From our mission

Gap Analysis Worksheet

CULTURAL TRAIT	IS NOW	SHOULD BE	GAP
1. Performance is:			
2. Good performance is:			
3. Success is:			
4. Information is:			
5. Management is:			
6. The future requires:			
7. People are managed:			
8. Resources are allocated:			

TOOL B: Self-Assessment: Strategies for Building TEAM Commitment

Instructions: Appoint a recorder and timer for your group. You have _____ minutes in which to complete this activity.

Objectives:
1. To teach team members the value of building team commitment
2. To develop strategies for building commitment in the team

Supplies: team commitment survey

Time requirement: 1 hour

Step 1. Jot down a few actions, under each of the four strategies below, that your team now uses to build TEAM commitment.

Building clarity:

Developing proficiency:

Extending control:

Showing recognition:

Step 2. Have each member share his or her conclusions with the large group. Generate a list of commitment strategies that you will continue to use, develop new, or discard.

TOOL C: **What Do We Expect from Our Team Leader?**

Instructions: This self-assessment tool is to be used when the team leaders wants feedback from team members about their performance, to strengthen leadership in the team.

Objectives:
1. Provide an opportunity for the team to practice giving constructive feedback.
2. Assist the leader to understand what the team believes are leadership behaviors that help or hinder the team in the accomplishment of its work.
3. Positive reinforcement of leadership actions that support group development and identification of areas for improvement.

Time requirement: 1 hour

Supplies: What Do We Expect? worksheet, flip chart, and colored markers

Method:

Step 1: Setting the context. The team leader or a designated outside facilitator sets the stage by asking team members to be open and candid in their reflections about leadership. They are encouraged to provide feedback that is both positive and supportive of the leader's strengths as well as areas for growth.

Step 2: Silent brainstorming. Team members are asked to reflect on their own expectations of leaders by answering the following questions:

• How does the leadership enacted in your home department compare with what you experience as a member of this team?

• Who was the most effective leader with whom you have worked? List the traits that stand out for you. Next to each trait describe why it was effective. (See worksheet.)

Step 3: Feedback exchange. Record on a flip chart the format described on the following page. Then ask each team member to report his or her ideas on leadership, collected from the responses to the previous brainstorming questions.

Once all ideas have been collected, the leader and team members review each item and select three areas of strength. Discussion should focus on why these leader actions assist the team in completing its work. Circle these traits in red.

Next review the list again. What areas of growth might the team leader pursue in the future? Team member discussion should become more specific on why team members need a certain kind of behavior from the leader. How will it support the team member personally or improve the team's efforts? Circle these items in green.

Step 4: Validation and improvement. The team leader summarizes the feedback received. Both strengths and opportunities for improvement are identified. The leader identifies actions that will be taken to improve leadership and sets a date for reevaluation with the group. If the feedback is largely overwhelming to the leader, the leader commits to review the information with his or her coach and to get back to the team at the next meeting with action plans for improvement.

What Do We Expect from our Team Leader		
LEADERSHIP BEHAVIOR	**IMPACT ON ME?**	**TEAM IMPACT?**
1. Admits mistakes	• I can learn from my mistakes	• We correct errors befire they get out of hand.

Four Tips for Managing Conflict in Work Teams

Consider the following steps when you anticipate conflict-prone agenda items:

1. *Disseminate a full agenda early.* This allows group members to prepare for all discussions before the meeting. Consider ordering the agenda so that the least emotional issues are taken care of first.

Outcomes:

Provides a focus to the meeting

Allows enough time for real discussion

Desensitizes the group to the more emotional issues

2. *State the team accountabilities for dealing with conflict.* Identify the negative consequences of destructive conflict. Reinforce team norms. Consider developing a conflict management guide, if you have none in place, that outlines what team members believe about how they will work together.

Outcomes:

Group recognizes dangers of destructive conflict and self-corrects

Behaviors of constructive conflict management displayed

3. *Script the meeting ahead of time.* Identify the outcomes you wish to achieve for each agenda item and the strategies you will use to assist the group in getting there. Use a more experi-

enced leader to help you identify both strategies and anticipated outcomes. Understand your own "hot-buttons" about the issues at hand and think about how you will prevent them from interfering in the resolution of team conflict. (*Hint:* If you feel strongly about the issue you might ask someone else to lead the discussion or temporarily step down from your team leader role, announcing to the group you wish to participate as a member. In this way, you do not risk imposing your beliefs as a leader on the whole team.

Outcomes:

Expected outcomes of the group's work conveyed clearly

Processes applied to foster cooperation and openness

Conflict planned for and managed

4. *Manage the physical environment (seating, room size, and tables).* This strategy is often overlooked or minimized in its importance to group effectiveness. Preparing the room so as to maximize dialogue and minimize subgroup can be very helpful.

Outcomes:

Coalitions seated in neutral positions

Power differences neutralized

Networking/team building emphasized

TOOL D: A Self-Assessment: What Do I Believe about Conflict?

Instructions: As a member of a team, you are bound to encounter conflict, which must be managed if your team is to be successful. Conflict management causes us to think (or perhaps re-think) about our professional roles, ourselves, our values, our relationships, and our organization. The statements below, which you are to complete, should help us get started on this. Try to be as candid as you can in making your responses. After you have finished with this form, be prepared to share your conclusions in discussions with other team members.

Objectives:

1. Assist teams to assess their conflict management methods for effectiveness
2. Provide an opportunity for team members to express satisfaction or dissatisfaction with conflict management methods used in the team
3. Provide the opportunity for team members to explore how personal experiences contribute to beliefs about conflict management

Time requirement: 90 minutes

Materials: "Focusing On Conflict" Handout, 9 Flip Chart Posters and magic markers.

Method

1. *Reflection.* (20 minutes)

Have participants silent answer the 9 questions on the "Focusing On Conflict" Handout. While they are working, the team leader or facilitator creates nine "posters" by taping together four flip chart sheets to make a large poster. Tape each of the nine across an available wall. Print one of the nine focus questions at the top of each poster, using a different colored magic marker.

2. *Compilation* (25 minutes)

As team members complete their self-assessment, have them record each of their answers on the appropriate poster. When everyone is done, invite the team to mingle and review the comments on each poster, in preparation for a discussion of the team's conflict management beliefs and practices.

3. *Dialogue and Strategies For Improvement* (45 minutes)

Once everyone has recorded their responses, lead the team in a discussion of each poster. Ask the following questions about each poster:

- What Are The Predominant Themes For Each Question? Are Several Of The Answers Similar? Can You Consolidate These Into One Statement?
- How Do our Beliefs About Conflict Influence our Behaviors In This Team?
- How Do Differences In Personal Approaches To Conflict Management Help or Impede Conflict Management In This Team?
- Do We have Some Predominant Ways of Managing Conflict? Are They Effective?
- How Does Our Organization's Response To Conflict Influence The Way We Behave In Conflict Situations?
- What Do We Want To Do With This Information?

Focusing on Conflict

1. My biggest achievement on this team has been:

2. If I could redo one aspect of my position on this team I would:

3. If I had to state what the two most important things about conflict management in this team are, I would say:

4. My definition of a team-related conflict is when:

5. My biggest irritation when dealing with conflicts is:

6. My greatest satisfaction when it comes to conflict resolution is:

7. If my boss could change my conflict management style, he or she would:

8. If my peers could change my approach to conflict management, they would recommend that I:

9. If I could change the way our organization responds to conflict I would:

Identifying Milestones:
An Implementation Methodology Worksheet

Instructions: The practice of organizational discipline requires a consistently applied change methodology that specifies both steps to implementation and performance milestones. The following is an example of an implementation methodology worksheet that can be used for any change being considered by a team for implementation.

Implementation Methodology For City Hospital-Resource Management	
Step: 1.0	**Task:** Set expectations and prepare/orient Resource Management Systems Work Team
Duration: 6/96–9/96	**Task Objective:** To assure that work teams are prepared to achieve assigned outcomes for resource management.

Sub-task Number	Description	Outcome	Performance Measurement Tools
1.1	Key roles assigned and defined	• Leadership accountabilities	• Role Definitions & Expectations assigned
1.2	Guidelines established	• Workgroup expectations documented	• Accountability Guidelines
1.3	Knowledge base expanded	• Orientation to critical work achieved	• Resource Management Workshop and literature review**
1.4	Workgroups infrastructure in place	• Leadership and membership for work groups identified and in place	• Nomination, Validation And Appointment Process Defined

Team Consensus Worksheet

TEAM ISSUE	STEP 1 YOUR VIEWPOINT	STEP 2 THE TEAM VIEWPOINT	STEP 3 THE EXPERTS VIEWPOINT	THE DIFFERENCE BETWEEN 1 AND 3	THE DIFFERENCE BETWEEN 2 & 3

Peer Review: Task Force Recommendation to Team
DATE: July 4, 1996
TO: Women's Health Service Team
FROM: Chris Jeans, RN, Traffic Task Force Chairperson
SUBJECT: Recommendations for Commuting Alternatives

Background	In August the State will begin construction on a new highway and an overpass will be built across the north end of the Health Center's campus. The hospital has asked all service divisions to consider methods for lightening traffic on campus during peak periods.
Problem	We need to identify commuting alternatives and make a decision as to what would work best for women's health, as soon as possible.
Alternative 1: **Vanpooling**	Advantages: Disadvantages:
Alternative 2: **Flextime**	Advantages: Disadvantages:
Task Force Recommendation	

11 Team-Based Performance Evaluation

Those who sail the sea do not carry the wind in their hands.

Publilius Syrus

Everyone has experienced at some level components of performance evaluation. When people are employed one of the first expectations they have is that they will be evaluated at some point in their work experience.

Performance evaluation has historically focused on the activities and functions of the individual. Job descriptions and work standards have been defined against which individual performance is measured. Most performance evaluation reflects functional, activity-based, process-oriented criteria that indicate the relationship of individuals to the activities expected of them. These more functional action-based performance evaluation processes look at tasks, skills, activities, and specific relationships to determine the effectiveness of the individual in association with the expectations of the system. As a result, the focus of the individual's attention, as well as that of the organization, has been on the individual's functionality, skill exercise, and ability to fit within the group framework.

THE PROBLEM WITH INDIVIDUAL EVALUATION

Although there certainly has been much precedent for individual evaluation, there has been little evidence of its value. Most individual evaluation does discuss individual skills, abilities, talents, functional proficiency, man-

Performance evaluation has few supporters. Everyone associated with it knows that it measures little that is meaningful and produces few improvements in people or processes.

TEAMTIP 11.1

Changing from Process to Outcome

The format for evaluation changes with the focus on outcome. Some tips on changing mindset from process to outcome include the following:

- *Remove job descriptions as the basis for defining performance.*
- *Raise questions about the results of work rather than the process of work.*
- *Build the foundations of team-based performance measurement.*
- *Look for value in action instead of task-based functions.*
- *Challenge staff members to question everything about what is being done to see if it has value.*

In the new workplace the focus on value means reorienting to the content and character of work. The value equation drives all work:

$$Quality/Cost \times Time = Value$$

ual dexterity, and some elements of the individual's relationship to the group. What is not measured is performance within the context of value. Because value is an outcome-oriented notion and focuses on the effects of work, results are used as a means of evaluating performance. Results reflect the outcomes of the activities of performance and give evidence of the value of activity regardless of any other measure. The challenge with results-oriented or outcome-oriented performance evaluation is that little of individual evaluation translates well to outcome evaluation (Team Tip 11-1).

Although the organization can certainly look at the individual's relationship to performance outcomes, sustainable outcomes are the result of the integration of the activities of a number of individuals. Sustainable and comprehensive outcomes depend on the relatedness, the interface, and the relative contiguousness of a whole series of actions undertaken by a number of individuals. Outcomes are to drive the evaluation of performance. Value should be the foundation of the evaluation process. Evaluation mechanisms themselves must look not only at the individual but at the relationship of the individual's work to the work of others. When aggregated, they give evidence of comprehensive and sustainable outcomes. This understanding, however, changes the whole focus and meaning for performance evaluation.

No longer can performance evaluation simply be looked at in light of the efficiencies of process and the functional skills of individuals. Performance evaluation now must focus on the relationship between individuals, their activities, and the aggregation of those activities and their impact on sustainable outcomes in the delivery of service. This is especially true for health care.

Increasingly in the health care environment, payers, providers, and consumers are looking at what they get for their health care dollar. Several outcomes are reflected in this desire. First is the need to control cost and be clear that what is paid for service is reflected in the value one gets for that service. Second, payers, providers, and consumers look at the content of the service itself to ensure that the activities, functions, and processes associated with the activities result in the best level of service and the highest level of return. Third, there is a growing interest in the impact of health service on sustainable and continuous social health. Therefore a broad frame of reference is present as everyone looks at health as a community enterprise rather than simply a series of individual activities addressing the unique needs identified one person at a time. The composite and comprehensive health of the community (also known as the subscriber population) means a broader focus on the activity of health and a comprehensive source of measurement of the impact of those activities on the community as a whole. Each of these changes the focus of evaluation and enumerates a different set of expectations with regard to the evaluation of health care activities.

Team-Based Performance

As teams become the basis of work in the health care sector, the methods of performance evaluation shift. Teams become the basic unit of work and therefore the foundation for measurement of work and its outcomes. In team-based approaches the organization is not interested in the activities, effectiveness, or function of the individual but rather the outcomes of the team. Indeed, the team is obligated to be concerned with the work of the individual and the performance relationship that person has with the rest of the team members. As a result, two levels of evaluation exist: the team's internal evaluation of the relationship of each member to the others, as well as the individual's contribution to the work of the team. The second focus relates to the team's performance against the outcomes expected of it by the health care organization responsible for meeting the needs of its subscribers in the community it serves. Each focus is necessary to ensure that positive and meaningful outcomes are obtained and that team effectiveness is ensured within the context of doing its work.

The team's interest in performance evaluation is indicated in its relationship to each team member. The reverse is also true. Each individual has an obligation to evaluate the relationship she or he has to the team as a whole.

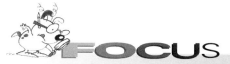

Value means getting the most for your dollar and obtaining the highest level of service from the provider. Value for the consumer is:
- A short, minimally intensive experience
- Healthful outcome
- Quality service
- Caring and responsive clinical staff members
- Good hotel services

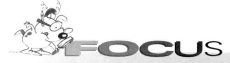

Three forces affect the future of health care:
1. Subscriber-based health services (managed care)
2. Advanced pricing of services
3. Building the continuum of services

That evaluation clearly emphasizes issues around relationship, conflict resolution, contribution, solution seeking, levels of investment in the work of the team, the fit between individual action and team process, the degree of consistent and continuous contribution of the individual to the team's effectiveness, and work processes. Each of these, and all of them together, reflect the relationship of the individual to the team. They should be a part of the continuous performance evaluation process that the team has within its parameters as it assesses its own functional proficiency, as well as its relationship to the outcomes to that it is directed. Criteria that reflect each of these elements or at least indicate the relationship of these elements to outcome will be a critical part of the performance evaluation process.

Here again, emphasis is not on the individual but the individual's relationship to the team. All measure of individual performance is a reflection of the individual as member of the team. What these elements of performance evaluation do, however, is recognize the individual contribution, the need of the individual to be recognized, and ties that recognition back into the individual's relationship to other members of the team who also need that same level of recognition.

Recognizing the Needs of the Individual

Simply because team-based approaches have been developed does not indicate that the unique characteristics and needs of every individual who makes up the team get lost in some amorphous team dynamic (Team Tip 11-2). Teams are groups of individuals gathered together for a common purpose, rendering their skills in a unique way to the benefit of the work outcomes that depend on the connected skill of all members of the team.

Performance evaluation is always a controversial dynamic in organizations. Exactly what should be evaluated, how evaluation processes should be constructed and conducted, and the role of the individual in the organization and in the team are the topics of much discussion. Each of these issues clearly affects an organization's approach to performance evaluation.

TEAM-BASED EVALUATION

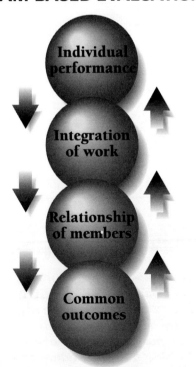

Individual performance

Integration of work

Relationship of members

Common outcomes

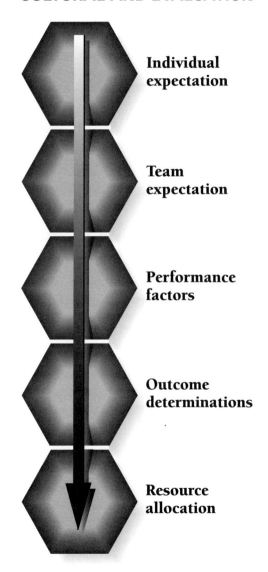

CULTURAL AND EVALUATION

Individual expectation

Team expectation

Performance factors

Outcome determinations

Resource allocation

TEAMTIP 11.2

Individual Recognition

Individual recognition is the foundation for building team-based relationships:

- *Team members acknowledge the value of each member of the team.*
- *Each member has a specific role to play within the team.*
- *Every member has a particular function with regard to other team members.*
- *Each member's contribution is enumerated in relationship to its value to sustainable outcome.*

The organization's culture supporting team-based approaches must also address the needs of the individual as a member of the system, just as it addresses the needs of the team and its contribution to the outcomes of the work of the system.

Every individual is intrinsically motivated by some composite of values and purposes that bring meaning to all of his or her endeavors. Extrinsically, the primary purpose of work at the individual level is to ensure that one can earn a satisfactory living and establish a satisfying quality of life. However, this extrinsic desire, while sufficient enough to keep people working, is not sufficient to keep them motivated. Therefore personal motivation demands more than simply meeting the extrinsic demands that bring people to the workplace (Box 11-1).

Therefore focusing only on the extrinsic factors does not adequately address the fundamental issues the individual brings to work, on which the advancement of work, improvement of quality, and sustaining involvement in that work require. Intrinsically, individuals at some level of function

BOX **11-1**

Individual Motivation

The ability to keep people involved and invested in their work depends on the organization's ability to allow the worker to fully participate in decisions about his or her work. As well the worker expects:
- Clarity about the expectations of the work
- Freedom to make decisions related to the work
- Involvement in policy decisions affecting the work
- Generation of information affecting the work
- Honesty regarding the goals of the organization
- Sufficient support to do the work

BOX **11-2**

Ensuring Autonomy

Each professional needs a level of autonomy to be fully invested in his or her work and to contribute to the goals of the system. There are central obligations on the part of the system necessary to ensuring autonomy in decision making:
1. Each worker knows the parameters of individual decision making.
2. The worker is expected to make independent decisions.
3. Each decision reflects the relationship it has to obtaining team outcomes.
4. Each decision maker has the skills necessary to make good decisions.
5. Every decision maker knows the "fit" of his or her decisions with those of other team members.

have a natural inclination to advance their interest, use their creativity, develop their skills, and apply their talents in a way that optimizes what they have to offer. Research has indicated that the primary rewards such individuals are looking for is their impact on outcomes (their effectiveness) and the autonomous sense that their work has impact and makes a difference.

This need for autonomy is perhaps one of the most difficult issues to address in team-based work systems. Becoming a member of a team does not in itself create an amorphousness, lack of identity, or merger of individual identity into a broader-based team character. Individuals remain individuals. Their need for self-satisfaction, self-determination, and ability to make a difference remains intact regardless of their relationship or the interactions they may have with others. A part of the obligation of work is the assurance that these unique individual characteristics do not get lost in team performance but are incorporated in the expectations for team-based evaluation. This need for an internal locus of control and individual sense of value must in some way be supported by the organization and its processes (Box 11-2). Each profession and its professional members identify themselves within the context of their discipline. Creating an interdisciplinary multifocal work group does not force individuals to lose their identification and association with the professional group through which they entered into the health care arena. Membership with their profession empowers them to exercise the work of that profession and gives them a specific identity, as well as a collective affiliation.

Professionals identify themselves with their profession. At work that identity does not disappear. The individual expects the identity to be honored, not diminished.

One of the serious flaws in most organizational renewals in health care is the diminishing value placed on professional identity in the interest of building teams and creating a new work relationship. This relationship cannot be obtained at the expense of professionals and their individual identity in relationship to their work. Professionals are faithful to their work, not to the workplace.

In discussion about shared governance and empowerment processes, the autonomy of both the professional and the profession has been indicated as a critical measurement of motivation and satisfaction. This level of shared decision making, leadership, and indeed autonomy as a part of the professional's milieu has in the past decade increasingly been a part of the consideration of building organizational structure. Structures that support the autonomy of the professional, the unique contribution each professional makes, and the obligation of each professional to participate fully in decisions that affect her or his practice are fundamental constructs of the shared governance structure and its subsequent shared leadership and shared decision-making elements. Maintaining control over one's practice and influencing one's environment are considered central values of the professional's role. Those elements must also be incorporated into the process of measuring performance and ensuring effectiveness of the organizational system in support of the individual practitioner.

Competence is the life blood of any organization. It is exemplified by a clarity and tightness-of-fit between the work skills of the worker and the service needs of the patient. True competence requires that the outcomes

BOX 11-3

Techniques for Focusing on Outcomes

The focus on outcomes is a requisite for every role in the system. The following techniques make that happen:

1. Have staff members identify the results of their work rather than the activities they do.
2. Base performance measures on what happened, changed, advanced, or improved as a result of staff work.
3. Identify the team activities to which each individual contributes rather than simply an individual's actions.
4. Do regular quality reviews related to clinical pathways or protocols to determine best practices.
5. Have the team focus on the outcomes and "back into" problems with related processes.

of service be consistently achieved over time with the foundations laid for raising the standard of service.

Competence Value

Although the individual's needs must be addressed as a member of a profession, organization, and team, it is important to reflect on the limits of that as a foundation for performance evaluation. The satisfaction of the individual, level of sense of autonomy, and participation in shared governance are critical and affect the motivation of the individual. The ultimate value for the organization and the system is the impact it has on the consumer it serves. The true value of the system is the difference it makes in relationship to the service it provides in the community that it supports. Its fundamental value is evidenced in the outcomes it achieves (Box 11-3). These outcomes are most directly influenced by the competence of the organization in meeting its mission, achieving its goals, and making a difference in the community it serves.

In this frame of reference competence becomes critical. The individual has a serious commitment to his or her own skill, practice competencies, and ability to contribute to the outcomes of the work. This view is fundamentally individual and unique to the talents and skills the person brings to the activities of the discipline. The organization, however, is concerned with how those activities and skills, when combined with the requisite activities and skills of all those who have an impact on service, make the necessary changes that advance the work and the mission of the organization. Competency, therefore, has two components: that which relates to the individual's skills, abilities, and level of application, and that which evidences the system's ability to meet the needs to which it is directed. Because individuals are members of a system and have a broader commitment to the communities they serve, the priority for evaluation and for sustainability is in the outcomes that are represented in the aggregation of the work of all who make up the system.

In team-based approaches teams have specific activities, relationships, and values in light of the outcomes that they influence with those they serve. The patient populations that are served by specific teams should evidence specific outcomes in relationship to their needs, their request of the system, and their demand for health. Therefore team-based value is reflected in the tightness-of-fit between the activities and functions of the team (the competencies they bring) and the sustainable and continuous outcomes that are produced in relationship to those they serve.

Competency reflects the quality of work expended, the level of performance of individuals, the consistency of performance of individuals and of the team, and the interface of all activities around the team's obligation for service. In this frame of reference competency reflects both the individual's set of skills, commitment, and contribution, as well as the collective integration of all of those efforts within the team to meet the needs of those the team serves across the continuum of care.

Performance evaluation in this set of circumstances serves essentially two functions: the team is interested, first, in undertaking a reality check with regard to the performance of individuals and their relationship to each other; and second, in an evaluation of the outcomes of the work of the

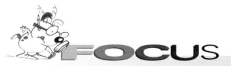

Getting teams together requires some specific activities at the outset of their formation. There is usually a series of activities that every beginning team should address:

- Rules of engagement
- Mission
- Meetings
- Processes
- Expectations
- Roles of members
- Accountability of the team
- Authority (power)
- Autonomy (decisions)
- Control (enforcement)
- Performance expectations

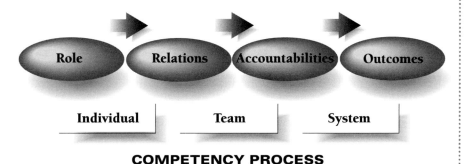

COMPETENCY PROCESS

Determination of competence is essential to the ability of the system to evaluate the outcomes to which work is directed.

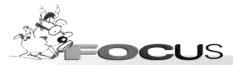

The system evaluates:
- *The team's work effectiveness*
- *The consonenance between the team and the expectations of the system*
- *The value of the team's outcomes*
- *The contribution of the team to systems value.*

The team evaluates:
- *Its functional proficiency*
- *The members' ability to work together*
- *The collective outcome of the team's work*
- *The ability of each team member to contribute to the team's work.*

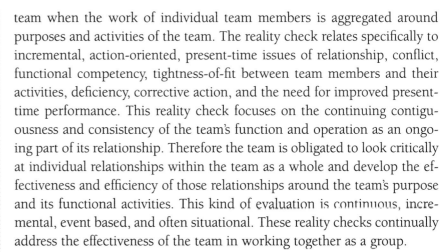

WORDS *of* WISDOM

Building teams is a process that changes the expectations for behavior. People cannot operate the same way in the team that they can individually. A new skill set is required to ensure that new behaviors can be expressed and be successful.

⁓

team when the work of individual team members is aggregated around purposes and activities of the team. The reality check relates specifically to incremental, action-oriented, present-time issues of relationship, conflict, functional competency, tightness-of-fit between team members and their activities, deficiency, corrective action, and the need for improved present-time performance. This reality check focuses on the continuing contiguousness and consistency of the team's function and operation as an ongoing part of its relationship. Therefore the team is obligated to look critically at individual relationships within the team as a whole and develop the effectiveness and efficiency of those relationships around the team's purpose and its functional activities. This kind of evaluation is continuous, incremental, event based, and often situational. These reality checks continually address the effectiveness of the team in working together as a group.

Team-based performance is continually unfolding. There is no evidence to date that teams ever arrive at a place of natural, normative, noncognitive resonance where all members of the team become actualized at a high level of interaction such that they represent a fluid and almost unconscious, naturally seamless group. While may occur in the future, most activities of the present are continuous and developmental and require frequent attention. Such reality checks become important, integral activities that facilitate the team's ability to identify its issues and concerns and to get at processes associated with naming problems, focusing on relationships, and addressing the psychological, personal, role-based barriers that exist between individual consciousness and the consciousness of the team. The psychosocial dynamics of building team-based processes require the team to confront, to address, to enumerate, to focus on individual as well as collective processes, and to be able, in a continuous way, to name the issues that impede the ability of individuals and teams to work within a collective framework. As has been outlined in previous chapters, much work is involved in building team-based relationships and consciousness, and techniques must be continuously applied through the reality check process to ensure the effectiveness of the team. Continually addressed in the reality check process will be issues around the ability to confront one's own behavior, conflict between personalities, skill differentiation, deficiencies versus differences, autonomy versus integration, discipline-specific requisites versus team-based activities, relational differences, and conflicts between and among various members of the team. All of these, while not encompassing all of the issues that will be confronted, clearly are continuous processes of a dynamic of team building. The reality check evaluation process requires team members to spend time in addressing these issues.

The second component of performance evaluation, the team's assessment of its activities against expectations or outcomes for those activities, is much broader and requires a more formalized, structured process of evaluation. It is here where the quality improvement processes and evaluation mechanisms have an important significance to the system. The mission and purposes of the organization are exemplified in the outcomes of the activities of the team. Therefore the team-based approach to evaluating

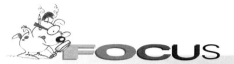

FOCUS

New behaviors inculcated into the team are:
- *Dialogue*
- *Managing differences*
- *Diversity sensitivity*
- *Outcome orientation*
- *Conflict processes*
- *Group processes*
- *Use of quality improvement tools*
- *Personal and group awareness processes*
- *Work and relationship evaluation*

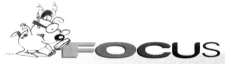

FOCUS

Evaluation skills are essential to the effectiveness of teams. Evaluation is driven by outcomes and forms the format for measurement. Members must be able to:
1. *Suspend personal judgment*
2. *Listen carefully to critical process*
3. *Focus on the results of a task, not the process alone*
4. *Focus on teamwork, not individual activities*
5. *Tie each person's actions into the expectation of the team*
6. *See every element or action as a part of a whole from the perspective of the whole*
7. *Problem solve together using formal methodology*

its functions and activities against its standards, critical paths, best practice measures, quality measures, and outcomes measures becomes the critical work of team-based performance evaluation. These processes are imbedded in the activities of developing a team-based approach to reviewing team performance and evaluating its effectiveness.

BEGINNING TEAM-BASED MEASUREMENT PROCESSES

At the team level the foundations for performance measurement must be clearly apparent to each team member and to the team as a whole. The team-based measurements must be a consistent part of the expectations of performance for all members of the team. Performance expectations relate predominantly to the team's ability to fulfill the obligation to which it is committed. Furthermore, the team is obliged to ensure that its activities contribute in an ongoing way to the work of the organization and the outcomes to which it is directed.

Each team member must understand just what will be measured and what the foundations for measurement are. Therefore the team should consider the following issues as it begins to establish a basis for ongoing measurement and performance review:

- The team members agree on what it is they intend to measure.
- The team is clear about the necessary frequency of measurement.
- The team is clear on the criteria used for measuring performance.
- The team develops and agrees to the processes, methods, and tools used for evaluation.
- The team is clear about the fundamental questions that are being addressed in measuring its clinical performance and its service expectations.
- The team has sorted out who will be involved in the measurement process.
- The mechanics of outcome evaluation have been clarified by the team.

For the team to agree on what it intends to accomplish, it must use good process. The discipline of method is required for good processes. No longer should team meetings be conversations and discussions. Rather, they should reflect good dialogue around a disciplined process that leads to an applicable outcome.

- The kind, character, and frequency of data review are identified by the team.
- The processes and mechanisms associated with corrective action are identified in advance by the team.

The above activities form the foundation on which performance measurement will be built. Unlike individualistic performance evaluation of the past, performance of the team is tied directly into the expectations and outcomes of the activities that the team members are involved in. The team's obligation is to make a difference with regard to those it serves in relationship to the expectations the organization has for the team. Therefore all team-based evaluation is tied specifically into performance measures, outcome measures, activity assessments, and the generation of data and corrective action that addresses the team's response to what it is evaluating. Team-based evaluation will be frequent, continuous, ongoing, and developmental. In team-based performance evaluation there is very little end-of-year or annual evaluation emphasis because to do so would wait too long to be able to make the incremental adjustments and changes necessary to make sure that the team is effective. Therefore team-based performance evaluation is a much more frequent activity that is integrated into the functions and roles of the team as it undertakes its work over time.

Measurements of progress against clinical objectives and performance expectations should occur at the same time as evaluating the team's effectiveness. The internal and external relationships help establish the team's focus on building relationships around the expectations and outcomes to which the team is directed. This takes the team's attention away from simply focusing on personal or individual issues and looking at individual performance and functions in light of the expectations the team has for outcomes.

Clinical Measures

The predominant framework for measuring a health care team's behavior will be clinical measures. Critical paths, clinical criteria, standards of prac-

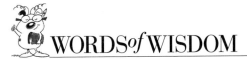

WORDS*of* WISDOM

Performance evaluation has an impact on future performance and improvement.

Team focus helps members see the whole, not just the parts that are theirs.

BUILDING BLOCKS FOR TEAM EVALUATION

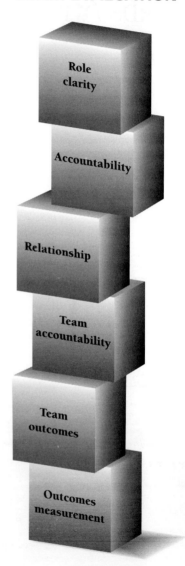

Role clarity

Accountability

Relationship

Team accountability

Team outcomes

Outcomes measurement

tice, best practice criteria, clinical outcome measures, and performance outcome measures all serve as tools or vehicles of measuring the team's performance. The organizational objectives, pathway objectives, and priorities, as well as the team's own service objectives, are also part of the performance measurement process. Each of these must be integrated in a way that facilitates and affects the clinical practice of the team and the clinical expectations it has for service. All of these need to be integrated into an evaluation matrix that displays in a systematic and organized way each of the components of the evaluation process that must be addressed continuously and incrementally by the team. These elements of performance are part of the measurement devices that the team will focus on in the course of measuring its performance over time.

The quality improvement process when tied to performance evaluation (as it should be) also facilitates the generation of data that gives information to the team with regard to its performance against specified clinical outcomes that are identified as a part of the team's clinical process. This criterion for quality improvement unfolds out of the team's

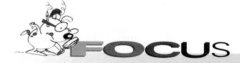

FOCUS

Differences in Performance Factors

Individual Performance	Team Performance
• Functional proficiency	• Member contribution
• Technical competence	• Role fit
• Process activity	• Team outcomes
• Individual work activities	• Team critical process
• Individual performance review	• Team performance review
• Individual reward determination	• Team rewards

approach to providing the activities associated with its individual critical paths, clinical processes, or best practice framework. These functional pathways provide the framework within which the clinical team identifies the relationship of each member to the processes for which he or she is individually responsible and ties each of these discipline-specific processes together to the patient or service outcomes to which all team members are committed.

Because of the amount of development that has occurred on constructing clinical processes, clinical paths, and best practices, there are a number of tools available to teams that focus on the relationship between the clinical process and specific clinical and performance outcomes. Most health care institutions have made considerable progress in developing critical paths, care maps, best practice processes, and protocols. Each of these can be used specifically as a part of the team-based performance evaluation process in light of the outcomes anticipated in each patient pathway within which clinical processes have been developed.

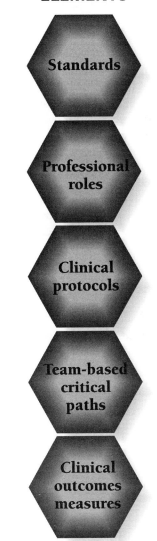

CLINICAL EVALUATION ELEMENTS

Standards

Professional roles

Clinical protocols

Team-based critical paths

Clinical outcomes measures

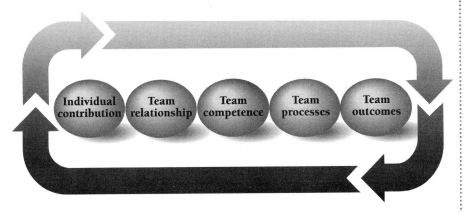

EVALUATION INTEGRATION

BOX 11-4

Timing Affecting Performance Review

Team-based performance review is not driven by annual events. It is a continuous process that is tied specifically to the achievement of clinical outcomes. Three factors affect timing of reviews:

1. Sufficient aggregation of patient cases within a clinical path providing adequate data for review
2. Any issue or event not in context with the standard or performance expectation for the clinical process
3. Changes in team expectation, behavior, or processes requiring team evaluation

Evaluations are not disciplinary processes. They are reviews of status and circumstance. They require a moment of analysis and synthesis and decisions that will affect the outcomes of relationship and work. Evaluations assess "fit" between structure, process, and outcome. That is the context within which they should be viewed.

Measurement Requisites

Although there are processes and mechanisms available for performance measurement against clinical processes and outcomes, there is no specific formula as to when measurement should occur. The criteria of measurement should include the time frame for that measurement as it relates to how data is generated, how it is communicated, how it is reviewed, and how well it is designed in a way that is useful to the team (Box 11-4).

Teams need to measure in a continuous and incremental way. While they can establish quarterly, twice yearly, and annual measurement times depending on the issues, the need for corrective action, the adjustment in the clinical process, and the functional focus of the team there may be a number of different measurement processes that are aligned at different times and for different reasons during any given year. More frequent evaluations of criteria adjustment, skill development, performance deficits, and incremental outcome problems may be required in between the more established, recognized formal evaluation times.

The following guidelines should be used in making decisions about when to evaluate the team's performance:

- Measurement should always take precedence over the need for corrective action as close to the corrective action as possible.
- Small units of measurement should be undertaken regularly to define smaller successes on which the team can build. The team needs to measure its successes along the way just as it needs to enumerate the successes over the long term.
- The incremental measures of success, corrective action, or performance improvement need to interface with the regularly scheduled matrix of evaluation and performance criteria.
- Included in the team's evaluation should be its review of its evaluation processes.
- Although outcomes and performance are critical, reviewing the mechanisms, methodologies, and techniques of such processes is also an important part of effective performance measurement.

- Careful attention should be paid to the way data is constructed and collected so that it can be done easily, simply, and with value. Highly complex, statistically difficult, and detailed evaluation processes often yield little value to the clinical practitioner in a way that can be readily responded to with understanding and commitment.

The matrix for performance evaluation in the areas related to patient or service outcomes should also indicate the time lines expected for various components of the evaluation so that the formal, quarterly, half-year, or annual processes are enumerated as a framework for the subprocesses that might take place daily, weekly, monthly, or bimonthly. A matrix that measures the component of measure, who conducts the measure, the sources or tools of measurement, the frequency of measurement, and the outcomes of that measurement can become a simple, easy-to-use tool that helps the team stay focused and gives the team a template within which it can unfold its measurement process.

Teams should also be able to access existing data that is continuously generated within the system in a number of different settings (Team Tip 11-3). Some of this data can be very valuable and assist the team in focusing its own activities and review processes without having to develop additional performance tools to do so. Examples of quantitative data that is collected in systems that may be of value to teams include the following:

- Quality assurance data records
- Service records
- Tracking inventories
- Order-entry records
- Past budgetary historic data
- Vendor and equipment service records
- Departmental-based quality measurement data
- Patient or customer satisfaction surveys
- Organizational and department audits
- Project evaluations
- Employee opinion surveys

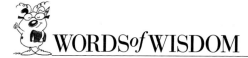

WORDS *of* WISDOM

Improvement is the outcome of all evaluation!

All team reviews should have an identified time line. Time provides the discipline that requires results be measured or obtained. No evaluation process should be undertaken without clear and specific dates when the process is reviewed or concluded.

TEAM**TIP**   11.3

Data Availability

In team-based approaches all data necessary to obtaining or sustaining outcomes should be available to the team. In team-based approaches the role of leadership is to see that the team has all the information it needs to thrive and advance the work of patient care.

- Employee satisfaction surveys
- Retention turnover figures
- Length of stay and other patient-based data
- Meeting minutes and other logs of quality process
- Calendars of events and agendas
- Incident reports and workers' compensation reports

Although this list is not exhaustive, it does give the individual some idea that there are a host of already present data tools that, when combined with individual team-based or pathway-based evaluation criteria, can provide a composite of information that is useful in undertaking team-based performance evaluation.

Creating Process Formality

A framework for continuous team-based performance review must include the focus on a process or methodology template that makes it possible to

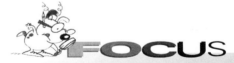

FOCUS

Good Methods for Team Evaluation

Teams must use all the tools that are commonly available for evaluating their work and its outcomes. Following are some of the common tools used for team evaluation of its work:
Focus group process
Surveys
Report cards
Check sheets
Logs
Histograms
Pareto charts
Trend, run, and control charts

facilitate good evaluation. Every team can design methodology that fits its specific characteristics and the focus of that which it is evaluating. However, the methodology selected should be consistently applied as a vehicle for development of the team members in the skills around continuous outcome evaluation.

The quality movement has provided us with many tools that help formalize the process of outcome-driven measurement. Using processes that relate more specifically to the quality improvement dynamic of the organization helps not only integrate the two components-team-based process and outcome evaluation—but provides a stronger framework for continuous evaluation.

The connection between process improvement and team-based performance evaluation provides a construct within which performance evaluation can be more clearly articulated. The greatest payoffs that result from a focus on process improvement are evidenced in its commitment to the creation of effectiveness, which is doing the right thing; efficiency, which is doing things correctly in the appropriate time with a minimum use of resources; and adaptability, which is responding in a timely and appropriate fashion to the changes and adjustments necessary in the system.

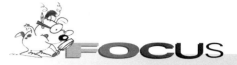

Three of the Best Toolbooks Around

The Health Care Manager's Guide to Continuous Quality Improvement, *by W. Leebov and C. Ersoz (American Hospital Publishing, Chicago, 1991)*

The TEAM Handbook, *by P. Scholtes et al. (Joiner Associates, Madison, Wisc, 1992)*

Continuous Improvement Tools, *volumes 1 and 2, by R. Chang and M. Niedzwiecki (Richard Chang Associates, Irvine, Calif, 1993).*

Bibliography

Beckham D: Building the high performance accountable health plan, *Healthcare Forum Journal* 37(4):60-67, 1994.

Bell C: *Managers as mentors: building partnerships for learning,* San Francisco, Berrett-Koehler, 1996.

Blanchard K, Carlos J, Randoph A: *Empowerment takes more than a minute,* San Francisco, Berrett-Koehler, 1996.

Center HI: *The medical outcomes and guidelines sourcebook,* New York, Faulker and Grey, 1994.

Crystal B: The 360 degree assessment, *Healthcare Executive* 9(6):14-17, 1994.

del Bueno D: Evaluation: myths, mystiques, and obsessions, *Journal of Nursing Administration* 20(11):4-7, 1990.

Dunham N, Kindig D, Schultz R: The value of the physician executive role to organizational effectiveness and performance, *Health Care Management Quarterly* 19(4):56-62, 1995.

Flynn AM, Kilgallen ME: Case management: a multidisciplinary approach to the evaluation of cost and quality standards, *Journal of Nursing Care Quality* 8(1):58-66, 1993.

Kotter J, Heskett J: *Corporate culture and performance,* New York, Free Press, 1992.

LaPenta C, Jacobs G: Application of group process model to performance appraisal development in a CQI environment, *Health Care Management Review* 21(4):45-60, 1996.

Lawler E, Mohrman S, Ledford G: *Creating high performance organizations,* San Francisco, Jossey-Bass, 1995.

Lombardi D: *Thriving in an age of change,* Chicago, Health Administration Press, 1996.

Longo D: The impact of outcomes measurement on the hospital-physician relationship, *Topics In Health Care Financing* 20(4):63-74, 1994.

Ludemann, R, Lyons W, Bolck L: A longitudinal look at shared governance: six years of evaluation of staff perceptions. In Kelly K, Maas M (eds): *Health care work redesign: series on nursing administration,* vol 7, New York, Sage, 1995.

Luthans F, Hodgetts R, Lee S: New paradigm organizations, *Organizational Dynamics* 22(3):5-19, 1994.

Martin P: Evaluation of shared governance, *Journal of Shared Governance* 1(3):11-16, 1995.

Meyer C: How the right measures help teams excel, *Harvard Business Review* 72(3):95-103, 1994.

Omachonu V: Quality of care and the patient: new criteria for evaluation, 15(4):43-50, 1990.

Poirier C, Reiter S: *Supply chain optimization,* San Francisco, Berrett-Koehler, 1996.

Risher H, Fay C: *The performance imperative,* San Francisco, Jossey-Bass, 1995.

Schuster J, Zingheim P: *The new pay,* San Francisco, Jossey-Bass, 1996.

Simon H: *Hidden champions: lessons for 500 of the world's best unknown companies,* Boston, Harvard Business School Press, 1996.

Swanson R: *Analysis for improving performance,* San Francisco, Berrett-Koehler, 1994.

Wilson T: *Innovative reward systems for the changing workplace,* New York, McGraw-Hill, 1995.

11 **TOOL**CHEST

TOOLA: Problem Team Member Leader Assessment Sheet

Planned Response or Action

All team leaders have team members who have difficulties adjusting, accommodating, or acting in a mature way within a group process. This is usually a part of the developmental cycle for group members. It is sometimes, hopefully rarely, a part of permanent individual problems with members of a group.

These kinds of problems demand specific response on the part of the leader to make sure that the leader is aware what kinds of activities need to be undertaken. A number of different instruments and tools are available that the leader can use to develop his or her ability and maturity in responding to problem members. This instrument serves as a simple tool to help organize and formulate the thoughts of the leader regarding response to specific kinds of problem behaviors.

Instructions: The format of this exercise is to provide a discipline for the leader to identify specific responses he or she might make to individual sets of circumstances. The purpose is to provide a critical framework for thinking productively about the kinds of reactions and responses the leader might make. The leader is advised to take these responses to a mentor or other leadership individual and explore the responses to test, validate, reinforce, or role play them before using them in the application of the leader's role.

Problem Team Member Leader Assessment Sheet

Team Member Problem: **Planned Responses:**

1. Member talks all of the time, drawing most of the attention to him or herself.

2. This individual is always involved in sidebar whispering or non-related conversations.

3. This person is action oriented and looks for decisions immediately before appropriate discussion has been held by the group.

4. This individual always makes a comment that is either unrelated or so far afield from the discussion it stops dialogue in its tracks.

5. This person consistently arrives late at every meeting.

6. This person consistently leaves early at every meeting.

7. This person have very infrequent or periodic attendance at meetings where he or she is expected to be present.

8. This person is consistently the group's funny person, always cracking jokes about the team's work or business.

9. This individual is consistently silent—has nothing to offer the group even though he or she is present.

10. This person has extreme difficulty in being concise, brief and to the point. Comments are usually always extended.

11. This person is either angry or consistently upset with the group and sees little value in its deliberations.

12. This individual complains constantly and can find nothing positive or productive to say in group meeting.

The above issues are representative of the number of kinds of problems persons might have as team members. The format of this exercise is to provide a discipline for the leader to identify specific responses he or she might make to individual sets of circumstances. The purpose is to provide a critical framework for thinking productively about the kinds of reactions and responses the leader might make. It is advised that the leader take these responses to a mentor or other leadership individual and explore them with them in order to test, validate, reinforce or role play them prior to utilizing them in the application of the leader's role.

TOOL B: Team Leader Observer Guidelines

The team leader must be aware of the behaviors unfolding in the team early in team development process. Looking critically and carefully at team members as they work together becomes a way of providing information to the team leader about the effectiveness of the team's processing. Looking at behavior is a critical part of ensuring team success. Five basic behaviors within group process must be observed: competitive, collaborative, task-oriented, planning, and action behavior. Each of these has an impact on the success of the group and the maturity necessary to meet the team's goals. The questions included in this instrument help raise issues regarding particular behavioral characteristics that should be identified within the context of the team.

Instructions:

Competitive behavior

- Is competition evident in the team?
- Can you as team leader identify the individuals who exemplify specific competitive behavior?
- How does the competition appear to be expressed by members?
- Is the competition due to competence issues or personality concerns?
- Does the competition impede the progress of the group in making its decisions?
- Can the competitive behavior be addressed individually?
- Is the level of intensity of the competition destructive to the group's integrity?

Collaboration

- Does the group appear to work well together?
- Are there individuals who have more clearly defined collaborative behaviors in the group than other individuals?
- Does the group reach consensus easily?
- Are there specific issues that affect collaboration and effective group communication?
- Is the group's skill level and maturity with regard to collaboration clear, or does it need further development?

Task-oriented behavior

- Is the group able to focus specifically on the tasks before it?
- Are the functional expectations of each member of the group clear to members?
- Are members performing consistent with their expectation and agreement?
- Are the outcomes expected of the group being achieved consistently over time?
- Does the group focus too much on activity and not enough on purpose and planning?
- Are the accountabilities of the team, as well as individuals, clear enough to enumerate performance?
- Has the team been successful in achieving specified goals?

Planning behavior

- Does the team have a specific plan identifying its direction and work?

- Does the team operate consistent with its planning activities?
- Is the plan consistent with the goals and objectives of the system of which the team is a part?
- Do team members clearly understand their role in relationship to the direction and plan of the team?
- Does the plan form the framework for the functional activities of the work of the team?
- Do team members reflect the plan in the achievement of their own achievement and professional goals?
- Is the plan updated and adjusted as information and circumstances demand change?

Action or work behaviors

- Does the team maintain a high level of commitment to its work activities?
- Is there clear evidence of energy and investment on the part of team members in their work and relationship?

- Do team members identify problems and issues of concern easily and readily with an attitude toward addressing them and responding to them?
- Are the activities of team members congruent with the expectations the team has for their individual performance?
- Do the activities of team members appear to be congruent with each other, fulfilling the collective goals of the team?
- Does a tightness-of-fit exist between the activities of the individual team member and the expectations of the team as a whole?

The above behaviors are representative of those necessary for effective team functioning. Leadership must remain aware of the impact of behaviors on the functional ability of the team. When those behaviors are not congruent or appropriate, leaders must address them immediately so that adjustments, refinements, shifts, and changes can be made to create a more effective team.

TOOL C: Team Coordination And Leadership Functions

Every team must be coordinated and led in a way that supports the work of the team and facilitates the direction of the team's activities. The role of the coordinator and facilitator of the team is critical to its success. Certain behavioral expectations are fundamental to the appropriate function and activities of a team coordinator or leader.

1. The leader always has the team deal with its own problems using a problem-solving process to seek solutions.
2. The facilitator anticipates conflict, identifies it early, and uses processes to resolve it.
3. The coordinator or team leader assists people in validating what went well in identifying the strengths and positive elements of the team.
4. The leader is honest and truthful in the presentation of all data, facts, and feedback.
5. The leader encourages the team members to be open, honest, and frank in their dialogue.
6. The coordinator or team leader is solution oriented and develops mechanisms and methods with the team that focus on solution, not simply on process.
7. Performance goals are used to evaluate the progress of the team at all times in its deliberation and its work.
8. The coordinator or leader is a generator of information, ensuring that the team has the resources necessary to make effective decisions.
9. The team leader uses the agenda and planning process as a means of anticipating and structuring the work and issues of the team over time.
10. Evaluation mechanisms are incorporated into the team's activities, and the team leader or coordinator uses these to measure the progress and effectiveness of the team's work.
11. The coordinator or facilitator accesses all resources and acts as a resource for the team at all times in the team's work.
12. The team leader provides for an appropriate feedback information mechanism to ensure that a cybernetic process continues with the team in all of its activities.
13. The team leader is aware of all changes or adjustments in information or data in advance of team deliberation to ensure that the team has the most current information available to it as it deliberates.
14. The team leader questions, raises issues, and casts out any process of decision-making effort or undertaking that appears incomplete or not consonant with the work of the group.

Leadership and coordination of the team requires being prepared to facilitate the work of the team, support the team, and provide opportunities for the team to be successful in fulfilling its purpose and doing its work. The above elements provide an opportunity for team leaders to be clear about specific expectations of coordination and leadership.

TOOL D: Becoming a Results-Oriented Person

Organizations are moving quickly from process orientation to results orientation. This shift requires a significant adjustment on the part of each individual in the organization. Because historically most of the values in an organization were related to process alone without a strong, clearly delineated relationship to the outcomes they produce, this shift creates "noise" in the organization.

Most of the personal noise in this shift relates specifically to personal adjustment to focusing on outcomes rather than activity. Everyone's activity should relate specifically to some meaningful outcome. The focus of this instrument is to assist the individual in challenging thinking between process orientation and development of an outcome mindset.

1. *Do I think of numerical goals or measures for the activities I am currently involved in?* An approach to using numerical objectives, measures, and standards indicators provides a framework for thinking about the value of one's work and processes. As one looks at data he or she is able to review clearly and critically the relationship between the activities and the results those activities achieve.

2. *Do I use short-term or long-term thinking strategies?* Short-term thinking is generally about specific functional activities. Long-term thinking focuses on the relationship between processes and the outcomes that are achieved. Most of us think in short-term measures. What have I just done, what procedure did I just complete, what work can I check off? Rarely do we spend time thinking of the long-term outcome to which

each of these activities relates. Outcome orientation requires this type of thinking.

3. *What kind of focus do I have in relationship to my work and its results?* Being focused on the day's work creates a mindset that impedes the ability to think comprehensively. The role of the professional is to tie processes together until they make sense when viewed as a whole. The role of focus is to help the individual understand the relationship between each incremental step and the comprehensive outcome to which those steps are directed.

4. *Do I have an accurate view of my contribution to the outcomes of work?* Often we see our work independent of the work of others. Rarely do we tie the activities of our performance with those of others upon which the outcome depends. In order to be able to work more effectively we will need to more clearly tie our own individual activities specifically to the activities of other team members so that we begin to see the results of the whole work in relationship to the outcomes of service.

5. *Do I really want to know my outcomes?* The fear of whether our work has value or not often prevents us from thinking about it in comprehensive terms. When we can check off our successes incrementally we can begin to feel that we are accomplishing something. However, when we have to look at all of our work collectively and begin to ask what difference it made in terms of outcome we may have less confidence and less assuredness that we have accomplished anything.

These five questions should assist the individual in undergoing a self-assessment around the readiness for results-oriented work and for the activities related to team process. Developing those become very critical to the individual's ability to focus appropriately on the results of work and to relate more specifically to the activities of the team.

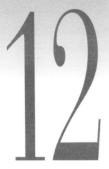

12

Evaluating the Team

Sustainable outcomes can never be obtained by individuals alone. It is the aggregation of the efforts of all upon whom the outcome depends that creates sustainability.

Tim Porter-O'Grady

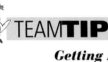

TEAM**TIP**   12.1

Getting Members to Think Outcomes

Creating a tightness-of-fit between process and outcomes is the work of team members and the major activity of leadership. Some tips that help:

- *In deliberations, always identify the anticipated or expected outcome first.*
- *When describing work, help staff members focus on the results of their efforts rather than the process.*
- *Help staff members tie issues or concerns to their impact on outcomes rather than be independent of them.*

Evaluating the team is a new process for most organizations. This process has a number of different characteristics from traditional individual performance review processes. The focus on team-based performance evaluation is specifically related to the team's ability to achieve outcomes. The activities of the team find their meaning and value in the relationship between them and the outcomes to which they are directed. A system is not well served by a performance evaluation system that does not tie action to outcome. This outcome-driven orientation distinguishes team-based improvement (Team Tip 12-1).

THE PLAN, DO, CHECK, ACT PROCESS

A number of approaches deal with team-based evaluation and tying performance to outcomes. Perhaps both the most effective and best understood format is the plan, do, check, act (PDCA) process. First identified by Demming earlier in this century, the PDCA process has become increasingly valuable as a context or framework for evaluation and processing improvement. It interfaces well with team-based performance measurement because what most of what teams are measuring are the outcomes of their work. Implementing the discipline of the PDCA model is a useful context within which performance evaluation can unfold.

Planning

The focus of planning is on a specific evaluative element or outcome and identifies all of those things that affect it, including patient expectations, clinical practice processes, problems, causes, inputs, outputs, solutions—almost anything that has an impact on identifying clearly what the issues are around which evaluation will unfold.

Imbedded in the planning process are questions that relate specifically to the level of understanding of the process that the team has in relationship to its clinical protocol or critical practice path (Team Tip 12-2). Questions that relate to the process itself serve as the focus for the planning activities.

- What are we doing?
- Where is the component of our activity?
- What are the process stages?
- For whom is it being done?
- What is the expectation of the providers? Of the consumers?

Planning does not mean that team members must know the endpoints of their work. Good planning means seeing the signposts of the organization's circumstances and its journey through them. Planning demands that the stakeholders be cognizant of the insights each has that, when joined together, create a complete picture of the work of the team.

TEAM**TIP**   12.2

Planning

The key to good planning is the ability to see the whole rather than just parts or pieces of any chosen strategy. The major initial activity is attempting to get the team members to see their efforts from the perspective of the whole rather than incrementally. Some techniques:

- Tie all process to mission and purpose so staff members see their work in the context of a larger agenda than simply doing the work.
- Name the outcome expectation first and place it on a flip chart so that it serves as the framework for deliberations.
- Grid the team responses around the purpose or mission so team members can make the connection between process and outcome.

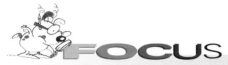

Planning means knowing your present status or condition as much as it means knowing your outcome. Some activities to define present circumstances are:

1. *Name anticipated outcomes and "back into" the reasons they are desirable.*
2. *Identify present issues or elements that make the outcome desirable.*
3. *Enumerate the role changes or behaviors that must be adjusted to make applying the outcomes appropriate.*
4. *Outline the activities of the team in relationship to the journey toward the outcome and the contribution of each member.*
5. *Determine the evaluation process, both incremental and outcome, to determine any adjustment.*

- What are the inputs necessary to make sure that the process unfolds?
- What tools and resources are needed?
- What are the relationships between each element of the process?
- What are the functional activities of each member of the team?
- How do the team activities interface?
- What does the approach look like?

In the process of planning you must be able to discern the difference between what your current processes are and what your best practices or ideal processes will or should be. Each clinical practice serves as a vehicle for improvement. The team looks at each of its clinical protocols as a vehicle for the improvement process and for making change in the team's activities. Therefore team members must understand collectively how their current processes work and what outcomes to which they are directed. All of the issues around the value of the process, how accurate it is, and what

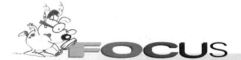

Planning means getting the team members to agree on a common set of expectations and a clear understanding of the contribution of each member:

- *Each team member is fully aware of the specific contribution he or she makes to the outcome.*
- *All team members are aware of the interaction their work has with the work of all members.*
- *There is tacit agreement on the part of each team member that any conflict will be worked out directly and immediately between the team members.*
- *Each member of the team recognizes that collaboration is critical to the team's ability to thrive.*

influences its effectiveness become an integral part of clarifying that current process. The critical path itself serves as a flow chart for enumerating the process clearly. In looking at the protocol, critical path, best practice, care map, or other tool the team uses for identifying its clinical process, the elements or the flow of services can be laid out clearly. This flow becomes the template for evaluating the effectiveness of various components of the process or the flow as a whole.

Clearly, once the flow is delineated, the individual obligations and activities of team members, the aggregated obligation of the team as a whole, is evidenced in examination and measurement of the flow chart and its components. Here also, the measurement and activity of a flow chart, the expectations that those activities lead as measured against the outcomes achieved, serves as a basis for measurement and analysis. The flow of processes uses a systematic and contiguous approach that provides data around the relationship between each step and the whole process. This blueprint serves as an architectural framework or road map against which each element and each component of the process can be evaluated in terms of its contribution to or its variance from the expectations of the process.

Based on the blueprint or map the team members can begin to identify areas of focus, variance from expectation, differences between the model and performance, and any other specific issues around performance against the map and its outcomes. In this way particular components of the process are identified on which the focus for improvement can occur. The process improvement ties into performance evaluation by enumerating the variance from expectation either in individuals' roles or the team function in a way that impedes the attainment of either the goals or the outcomes of a particular clinical process. Focusing on each of these elements of variance, change, or noncompliance in the process begins to configure team members around the interface of their activities in a way that affects the consistency and the continuity of all of the activities within the critical clinical care process.

Team members must always keep in mind that sustainable outcomes are dependent on the character and content of the relationship between the efforts of each team member. "Hero" and unilateral actions that fail to make the connection with the efforts of other team members are always an impediment to the team's ability to achieve sustainable outcomes.

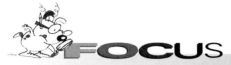

Variance from the standard or the protocol becomes an issue of serious concern to the team for two reasons that demand immediate evaluation and response:

1. The framework or baseline on which the team establishes its work depends on the consistency and constancy in the application of the activity that reflects them. Inconsistency always affects sound measurability.

2. The ability to replicate the activities of the team over time is an important part of validating the team's efforts. Good practice demands that the processes of the team be capable of being repeated and enhanced over time.

Out of this particular stage of analysis, looking at improvement, problem statements, and problem definition should be a major tool of identifying the variance or change that is required. Being specific, unilateral, and focused in defining the problem is critical. The problem should be defined in outcome terms. One should not simply identify the process. The provider will always want to link process to the outcomes to which it relates. Therefore any variance, problem issue, or concern within the pathway should be identified consistent with the outcome so that the focus of the team's work is on the fit between the process and the clinical outcome to which it is directed.

Once the process has been defined, the causal factors that relate to it become a critical part of the corrective action piece. The purpose of performance evaluation and team-based measurement is to undertake corrective action and bring consonance between the activities or actions of any one part of the team and the outcomes of the whole team. Therefore focusing on the fundamental and real-time causes of a particular issue or concern is a critical part of the problem-solving strategy. Once the roots of a particular problem have been defined it can create a way in which subsequent actions can reflect those activities that lead to facilitating the outcome. Facilitating the causal roots to problems is the inclusion of the patient's perceptions with regard to the impact of the process on patient satisfaction. Focusing on the patient or the consumer of the service helps focus the team on the issues of concern from the perspective of those who are recipients of the service.

Each problem identification, intervention, quality issue, and performance measurement element must ultimately lead to some solution that facilitates the outcomes of the particular clinical process. Solutions, while clearly identified with specific outcomes, should also be sustainable with regard to the outcomes.

Sustainable solutions are achieved when they facilitate the outcomes, advance practice, or raise the standard of performance to the expectations or beyond the expectations established for them. A number of solutions may fit any particular process, and it is appropriate for the team to identify the range of solutions that better fit and appropriately advance the outcomes anticipated.

The tools that can often be used for the planning process relate to the various components or stages of the planning process identified in the preceding paragraphs. The group process tools that are used are ones that best fit the definition of issues, the identification of problems, and the enumeration of processes associated with seeking solutions (Box 12-1). The following tools are helpful in this process:
- Brainstorming, focus group, individual interviews
- Care maps, critical processes, clinical process, protocol, flow charts, group process
- Histograms, surveys, log processes, check sheets, trend analysis
- Pareto charts, multivoting, decision matrixes, critical identification
- Cause analysis, affinity charts, cause and affect, tree diagrams, focus groups, force field analysis, nominal groups, relational diagrams
- Solution trees, decision matrix, brainstorming, priority setting, solution listing, cross-referencing

Every performance measure for the individual is a subset of measuring the performance of the team. No measure should be applied independent of the team. Outcomes are effective based on the team's performance. Any suggestion that individual performance acts independent of the team impedes team effectiveness over time.

BOX **12-1**

Team Process

Learning the techniques of team process is as important as any activity of the team. In the learning organization, the development of the staff members becomes critical to their ability to perform well. Some critical learning areas:
- Conflict processes
- Building relationships
- Continuous quality techniques
- Outcomes measurement
- Team member evaluation
- Skill set change

The action phase occurs only after the processes associated with action are clear to the members of the team. The team also recognizes the unique work framework it has and reflects that in the context of doing its work and achieving its outcomes. No action phase unfolds independently of relatedness to the results toward which it is directed.

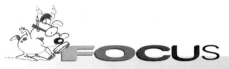

Doing

This is the action phase of the performance evaluation process. In the doing phase attention must be paid to the activities that address the deficits identified in the evaluation or planning phase. The evaluation simply has identified the activities and functions necessary to address the changes that are sought as the process unfolds. The action phase (doing) is where subsequent and substantive activity as outlined is undertaken by the team members to address the issues that they have planned to respond to. In this phase the variety of solutions identified in the first phase can be tested and experimented with to determine their appropriateness in application.

In the doing phase solutions are applied in a way that makes some measurable impact on the problem, issue, or deficit as identified in the planning phase. It is here essentially where experimentation is unfolding. There is still not enough clarity with regard to the appropriateness of response and not enough data generated at this stage to determine the tightness-of-fit between the response and the desirable corrective action. Sustainability is always the measure of effectiveness. If the change is outlined or the solution as applied has a sustainable impact on facilitating the outcome or improving the process, there is clear evidence that the solution chosen is appropriate. If it does not work, through incremental, regular, or periodic checks, process is then changed.

The doing phase of the performance/process evaluation dynamic means that every player has some obligation for the creation of a viable solution or outcome. All players' roles should be clear in terms of their contribution to the outcome and to the specific solution attempted to address it. In so doing, the specific and focused identification of those actions that do or do not contribute to advancing the outcome or improving the performance can be undertaken in an organized and consistent manner.

At this stage it is necessary to ensure that the action undertaken is consistent with the action planned. Often with performance evaluation, specific actions are identified as nonviable, not affecting outcome or playing a minimal role in advancing specific outcomes, and are therefore

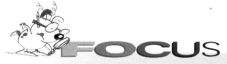

Each individual team member has an obligation to address his or her work with an eye on the fit between the team member's actions and those of the team and the impact on the patient. Sustainability depends on the high-level interface between the individual provider, the team, and the patient. The individual is always asking:

• How does what I am doing fit with my agreed-on activities?

• How are my activities reflected in the work of the team, and how do my actions fit?

• What do I see of my activities affecting the outcomes of the team?

• Are the clinical outcomes being achieved? How is the patient responding to the team's work?

dropped. The truth, however, is that often the application of action is inappropriate or not consistent with what was planned. The performance of the action may be subject to question. Careful consideration and analysis of the consistency of the action with the planned activity is a critical part of the doing phase on which good corrective action is based. Here again, the tightness-of-fit between the action and its impact on the outcome should be the best mechanism for measuring the effectiveness of the corrective action. The looser the fit between the outcome or expectation and the corrective action, the less likely that corrective action will have an impact on creating a sustainable or improved outcome. It can therefore be dropped, changed, or adjusted in a relatively brief period of time. However, the tighter the fit, the more sustainable the impact on the outcome and the more viable the activity. The doing phase produces the data on which these judgments can be made.

Inconsistent or noncompliant action or missed outcomes become an immediate point of performance evaluation for the team. If outcomes are not achieved or the processes are simply not fitting for a variety of reasons, a critical evaluation event is created to refocus the team on its efforts and their results. This performance evaluation does not wait for a particular time to unfold, rather it reflects a specific circumstance to which the team must respond.

The tools that can be used for activities related to the doing phase indicate an action plan. Activities and implementation processes include brainstorming, course correction, iterative adjustments, flow charting, force field analysis, logs, check sheets, and histograms. Team members should be familiar with the tools they need to use to make the process of evaluation more efficient and effective. These tools serve as an ongoing device for enumerating both the actions and their impact at the time they are being implemented and applied. In this way minor adjustments and corrections can be adapted in the action phase without having to repeat the cycle or become involved in broader assessment activities.

The check phase gives the team members the opportunity to measure where they are in relationship to what they have planned and whether the perceived activities and outcomes have a good tightness-of-fit. At this time adjustment and change are worked out and action is initiated in light of the team's work adjustments.

Checking

Checking in the PDCA cycle is tightly related to the process of performance monitoring and measurement. In the check phase the team evaluates the results of its activities, its solution seeking, and its processes against the outcomes achieved and the expectations identified for them. This check phase evaluates the critical efficacy and effectiveness of the corrective action as actually applied in relationship to performance.

The check phase should resolve many of the questions that were raised in the plan stage. Indicated in the check stage are responses to the questions that are specific and narrowly focused on the issues identified. The check phase should show the strong relationship between the causative factors and the solutions that were applied. In this way a sustainable foundation is established for corrective action and a tighter fit between the action and the outcome of the clinical process is established. In the check phase the following questions should obtain specific answers:

- Were the changes effective?
- Did they work?
- Is there a direct relationship between the improvement and the changes implemented?
- Is there a cost-benefit relationship between the two changes and their results?

- Has the continual and ongoing process been altered by the implemented changes?
- Does further refinement need to occur to create a better fit between the change and the expected outcomes?
- What further planning is indicated as a result of the implementation of the corrective action processes?

The tools used for the check section are reflective of the tools used in the previous plan and do sections. Those tools provide the information, documentation, and data that the check section depends on (Team Tip 12-3). In the check section additional tools that can be used are those that correlate the data, record and document the data in an organized and systematic way, and can be used efficiently to compare data and compare action responses. Therefore check sheets, logs, survey results, histograms, focus groups, trend analyses, force field analyses and Pareto charts are all tools that can be used in the process of assessment, drawing conclusions, and preparing to establish standardized responses to those actions that worked and related specifically to creating sustainable and appropriate performance.

Acting

The planning, doing, and checking phases are the initial and preliminary steps to the action phase. Action phase is where the positive, appropriate, and meaningful changes are implemented and incorporated into the ongoing activities of the organization. Actions establish the new baseline and new template for further evaluation, adjustments, and subsequent improvements in activity.

In the action phase the standardization or creation of new standards of approach is generated. In this way the improvements or enhancements are incorporated into the ongoing and usual work processes of the organization. Therefore the changes in the flow of activities or the critical path of activities are simply reincorporated into that flow and become a part of the baseline of observing, measuring, and monitoring that flow. Also, any standard of practice in other work flows where the particular change may also

---

TEAMTIP 12.3

Tools for the Check Phase
The tools used for this phase that are helpful to the team members in checking the viability of their efforts and work include the following:
- *Check sheets*
- *Experience logs*
- *Survey results*
- *Histograms*
- *Focus groups*
- *Delphi process*
- *Trend analysis*
- *Force field analysis*
- *Pareto charts*

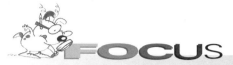

be beneficial can be incorporated into changing that standard as well. Generalizing those common activities to other pathways, critical paths, and best practices where it is appropriate helps diminish the amount of evaluation time and expand the applicability of certain analysis and corrective action processes.

During the action phase the new approaches and the new standardization must be communicated to all players on whom they have an impact. If a significant change alters the relationship within a team, between teams, in a pathway, or between pathways, it should be communicated through the normal communication pathways that are established for corrective action. Performance evaluation should always result in the advancement of performance, or the improvement of outcomes. Where that has an impact on others the benefit should be communicated effectively to them.

Many of these assessments require a change in practice, behavior, role, or relationship. Therefore the developmental or learning plan should in-

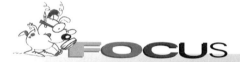

corporate these adjustments as a part of the ongoing development of the staff members responsible for implementing them. Where teams or pathway changes require a learned change behavior, learning processes and learning priorities should reflect the adjustments necessary to consistently achieve the outcomes identified by the improved practices. One of the most difficult elements of creating sustainable change is imprinting behaviors on the practices of the staff membes in a consistent manner. Often the lack of consistency in behavior and expectations creates most of the problems associated with implementing change. A good developmental and learning process that has in it its own implementation and evaluation elements helps address some of these issues.

Documentation and incorporation of the changes into the flow process, critical path, best practice, care map, and other documented approach to the regular flow of activities are important to ensure the standardization and incorporation of these into the ongoing baseline for any subsequent action. In the performance improvement framework, the new standard of performance, usually a higher level of expectation, should now become the baseline of expectation for measuring the performance of the team in relationship to its outcomes. In this way, the level of performance, the performance improvement process, and the quality improvement process all interface and link in a way that supports the growth, development, and overall improvement in the delivery of service and the satisfaction of the consumer.

At this stage performance evaluation and performance improvement must establish a new baseline for performance and begin the cycle all over again. The new standard of expectation now becomes the baseline for further performance refinement and enhancement. In this way looking at both performance and improvement becomes an integrated, correlated activity that not only advances the performance of individuals in the team but advances the outcomes and purposes of the team, the pathway, and the system. Incorporating the learning plan, strategic and tactical activities, and

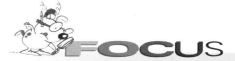

Standards now serve as the basis for enumerating and evaluating the action of the team and the activities of the individual. Several standard components serve as evaluative elements for the team:

- The critical path established for specific clinical processes
- The accountability elements for each member in his or her contribution to the critical path
- The performance expectations defined for each team member in his or her contribution to the work of the team
- The outcome expectations enumerated for each critical path or protocol for which the team is accountable

Documentation for evaluation purposes should be no different from and require no more paperwork than that used to document the work of the team and its clinical processes. The evaluation of teams and their members is imbedded inside every part of the work activities around the agreed-on processes and protocols developed together by the team members.

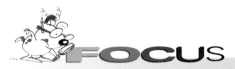

the individual and team-based performance grid serves now as the systematic mechanism for incorporating and developing team-based performance improvement as an ongoing part of the work in the organizational system. Developing the matrix that shows the relationship between each of these components and using it as a framework for identifying corrective action, evaluating performance improvement, and monitoring the rate of change and the compliance of activities with planned and expected outcomes provides the framework for the entire team-based performance evaluation mechanism.

Creating monitoring devices that begin to measure the new levels of behavior ensures a focus on just how much of the new behaviors become entrenched and incorporated as the new functional expectation for staff members and for the team.

The tools for the action phase that become a fundamental part of this piece of the PDCA cycle are monitoring tools, control charts, histograms, check sheets, skill checklists, trend surveys, satisfaction surveys, diagrams, and force field analysis. Each of these, when interfaced with the tools already present, provides a basis for ensuring that monitoring of behavioral changes, assessing the consistent application of these changes, and entrenching the change as the new baseline for performance occurs consistently at the team level.

The PDCA model for performance evaluation and improvement provides a framework, a cycle, a wheel, within which all of the activities of performance evaluation and improvement can be undertaken and located. It also provides a template or a framework within which the ongoing, continuous performance evaluation and improvement processes can be undertaken. While it is not the only mechanism for performance evaluation and improvement, it does provide a consistent and broad-based context that facilitates the formalization and ongoing incorporation of performance evaluation with service effectiveness, consumer satisfaction, care delivery, and outcome delineation.

GROUP PROCESS AND PERFORMANCE EVALUATION

All teams have a life cycle. The stages of team development have been identified from forming, storming, norming, and performing all the way through initiation to extinction. A wide variety of models have been used to identify the life process of groups. Performance evaluation and group life process are critical corollaries that must be addressed in any performance evaluation design and any group process assessment.

Every individual in a group affects the character and work of the group. In fact the group is whatever makes up the life of that group in each of its members. Group development, facilitation, leadership, and the movement toward outcome require an understanding of individual relationship to others and to group process dynamics. Increasingly, an understanding of the group and how the characteristics of individuals in the group work to facilitate it becomes important to the process of evaluating the effectiveness of the group.

In the life of any group the autonomy, status, independence, and identification of individual members are critical to their relationship to the group and their perception of other members of the group. Before groups can perform well together they must clearly enumerate what these perceptions are and the elements of their relationship one to another, as they begin to identify the interaction each will have with the other in the context of working within the group.

The organizational history and its culture have a clear impact on the viability, trust, and applicability of group process. An organization whose history is autocratic, hierarchical, and narrow in decision making will have a much more difficult time in creating effective group process than an organization whose history is engaging, horizontal, distributive, and empowering in its approach. The distance to travel toward group and team-based activities is considerable.

TEAM PERFORMANCE CYCLE

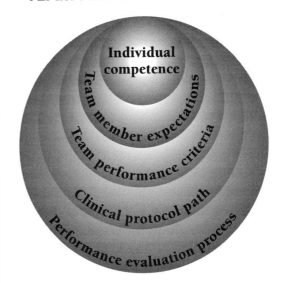

BUILDING BLOCKS FOR GROUP PROCESS

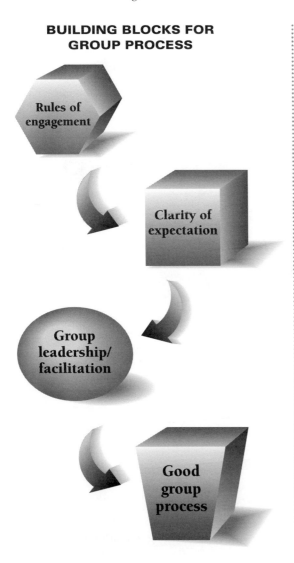

Rules of engagement

Clarity of expectation

Group leadership/ facilitation

Good group process

TEAM ADAPTATION

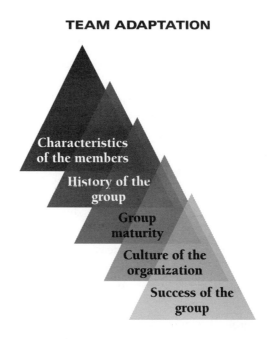

Characteristics of the members

History of the group

Group maturity

Culture of the organization

Success of the group

The higher variability of knowledge, understanding, and specificity of roles in professional discipline-oriented teams in health care creates a great barrier to the interface of developing a common knowledge and common intersection in team-based approaches. The differentiation of the disciplines has been critical to their identification and positioning. Therefore the disciplines come together to meet at the table to identify common approaches to delivery of service. The unfolding of their relationship challenges the imbedded differentiation of their knowledge base and will create problems for unification. Addressing those problems and their implication will be part of the initial stages of developing team effectiveness. This should also be a part of the initial performance evaluation activity as the team begins to assess its viability and its movement through its stages of development.

Because the culture does not yet have mature, well-developed point-of-service problem-solving and decision-making processes in place, much of the initial stages of developing performance evaluation processes will be related to the ongoing development of decision-making constructs for the team. Clearly, the evaluation processes at the outset of team-based formation will also look at the team's mechanism for decision making and the problems associated with getting team members configured around the decision-making process. The team's ability to perform together, to work together to resolve its relational and interactional problems, will be critical to early-stage performance evaluation activities regarding team development. Consistent performance cannot be obtained until the team members' basic relationships with each other have been plainly established and well developed.

360-Degree Performance Measurement

In team-based, point-of-service driven organizational systems, hierarchical, superior-subordinate performance evaluation processes no longer have meaning. Indeed they produce no viable results that sustainably affect performance and outcome over time. Therefore they have no purpose or value in a team-based performance system.

Every player who has an impact on the outcomes of the work of any other player must be involved in the life and activity of that individual. Therefore a part of performance review is evaluating the relationship of each player to other players within the set of relationships that define the outcomes, expectations, and performance of any given individual. The question as to who should be involved in individual performance evaluation of a team-based system is therefore easily responded to. Anyone who relates to or has an impact on the role of an individual in a team has an evaluation obligation and should be provided an opportunity to be a part of the evaluation of that relationship at any given time in the evaluation process. This 360-degree approach to performance evaluation and im-

ISSUES IN PARTNERSHIP

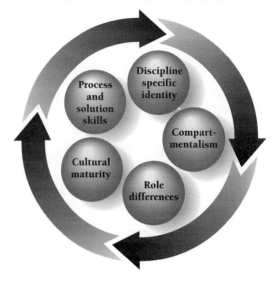

In the emerging whole systems approaches to structuring organizations, investment and ownership is necessary for thriving. The point of evaluation is the assurance that all people and processes are converging to fulfill the purposes and outcomes of the system. Evaluation mechanisms should support this expectation.

360-DEGREE EVALUATION

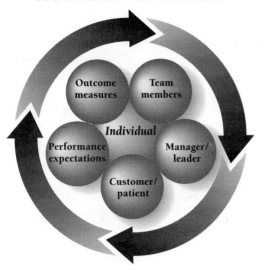

**TEAM
360-DEGREE EVALUATION**

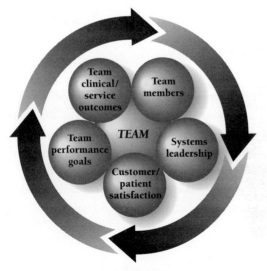

provement is a critical underpinning of team-based evaluation processes.

The team is always attempting to evaluate its effectiveness against the expectations for team performance. Therefore team members look at each other in relationship to their contribution to the team's role in obtaining those outcomes for which it has a defined level of expectation. Individual performance evaluation, then, simply relates the individual to the aggregated measures of performance. Every individual certainly looks at his or her role in light of the team expectations. In any review the individual looks at specific activities or functions that facilitated or resonated with the full team expectations. The reverse is also true. All team members look at an individual in light of the individual's fit with the aggregated activities the team expects. When there is variance, need for adjustment, or performance improvement, functional adjustment of that member's activities is needed to bring them in line with the team goal. The demand for adjustment can be exemplified by any one of a number of performance-related elements—the critical process, clinical plan, care map, best practice, or other format for delineating the team outcome.

Therefore three areas of team-based individual performance evaluation need to be articulated in the team's evaluation of its members and their performance against the expectations of the team with regard to outcomes: the individual's competence, team-based relationship, and exercise of accountability.

Team Member Competencies

Each individual professional or member of the team brings with him or her specific expectations for function and performance that his or her skill base, professional discipline, and role lend to the achievement of the goals of the team. As a result, standards, practices, routines, legal requirements, and other mandates of that member's discipline will be clearly articulated by the discipline for the team member before his or her membership on the team.

Whatever measures exist should reflect the unique character of the discipline's contribution, the clinical expectations for competence that the discipline provides for its members, and the team-based expectations for competence negotiated and delineated between and among the members of the team and the individual in the discipline. This serves as the foundation for establishing the specific, culturally driven, and professionally centered core competencies that will be continually examined and evaluated or expected of the team member when contributing to the work of the team. Clearly, competence should relate to the contribution the team member makes in the context of the performance expectations of the team. Each competency that is critical or core to the process of delivering service must be articulated in a way that can be understood by all team members and can be exercised by the individual professional working member who is expected to perform the competencies outlined.

Furthermore, the individual team member should also be evaluated within the context of his or her ability to identify shifts, adjustment, and changes in the core competence required to effectively perform as a member of the team representing that member's specific discipline or frame of reference. This individual should be able to anticipate questions, problems, and concerns with regard to his or her specific competency contribution. The individual should be able to organize functional activities, familiar and unfamiliar, within the context of the competencies expected of him or her. Where additional resources or insider information is required to refine the competency contribution, the individual is expected to obtain the information necessary to incorporate these into the baseline or standards of expectation for his or her performance as a member of the team.

All team members are considered able to function interdependently. The whole notion of independence or dependence is a specious one within team-based approaches. At some level of function the interdependencies define the parameters of the competencies that any one individual may express. There will be a number of options and opportunities to negotiate the application of specific competencies and the sharing of roles and functions with others who might also either develop these competencies or share them with the individual practitioner. Therefore this individual is able to consistently perform the core expectations and competency interdependently with other

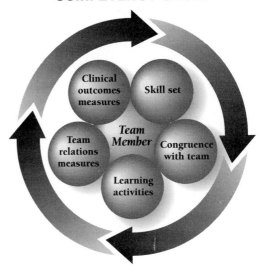

TEAM MEMBER COMPETENCY CYCLE

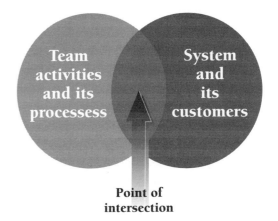

TEAM INTERDEPENDENCE

Every individual is expected to perform at or above the level of team expectation. Furthermore, all team members must give evidence of the ability to advance and grow in their practice and as team members. Good fit between all members and the expectations they have for each other in the achievement of outcomes is essential to the team's ability to thrive.

providers and practitioners. There should be clear evidence of the interface between the individual competencies and skills and the collective demand for competence regarding the outcomes to which each role is directed.

Within the framework of individual competencies in a team format there is an expectation on the part of the team members that the individual will

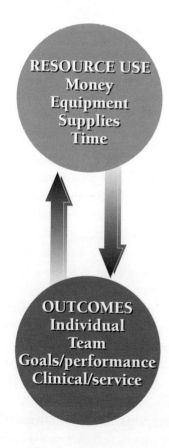

RESOURCE-OUTCOME INTERDEPENDENCE

RESOURCE USE
Money
Equipment
Supplies
Time

OUTCOMES
Individual
Team
Goals/performance
Clinical/service

give evidence of the ability to adapt, to adjust, and to shift in a fluid and flexible way. Mobility is the measure of viability of team membership. The need to maintain that mobility and fluidity will be important as the character, content, functions, and activities of providing health services shift as the locus of control for health care shifts and as the point-of-service becomes the more critical and appropriate locus for decision making. The relationships, intersections, adjustments, changes, critical paths, and continuum issues that affect the unfolding of individual and team-based practice will require a high level of flexibility and adaptability to change. Therefore the team has a right to expect of the individual an attitude, a performance viability, and a level of willingness to embrace and engage change and to incorporate that change into one's own practice. The ability to seek support and to use it where appropriate should also be enumerated in a performance evaluation process. A positive disposition to the processes of change and the adaptability of new skills and expectations in roles should also be a part of what is anticipated and expected in the individual team member's roles and should be evaluated by the team as a whole.

Of equal importance is the ability of the individual to be organized, to be systematic, and to manage time effectively in delineating his or her role. Each team member should be able to give evidence of good organization, sound time management, and the structuring of his or her routines in an appropriate and timely fashion. Increasingly in team-based approaches, tightening of resources and increasing demands for outcomes create an emphasis on tightly defined time management. It is therefore appropriate for team members to expect of team individuals the ability to organize and use their time wisely and efficiently. Good time management should be a part of the team's evaluation of its individual members.

Team Member Interdisciplinary Relationships

The team is a human group. Therefore it is subject to both the foibles and facilities of team process. The development of processes associated with building effective and meaningful teams takes a considerable period of time.

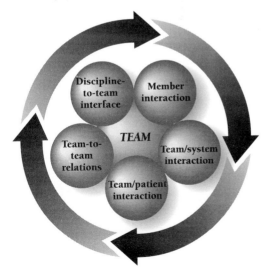

TEAM-INTERDISCIPLINARY RELATIONSHIP CYCLE

Through the use of well-devised and well-defined techniques and methodologies, that time frame can be tightened. However, an ongoing monitoring and assessment of the interpersonal relationships between members of the team will be a critical part of ensuring its ongoing effectiveness.

The ability of the individual to interact well with other team members, get along well with them, and be enthused about his or her relationship with them is an important part of the team-based development process. There should be evidence of the effective ability to interact well with people, to confront difficult situations, to problem solve, to face conflict where it occurs, and to use the techniques and methodology for resolving conflicts without heightening interpersonal anxiety. Each of these elements and skills will be necessary for effective team-based functioning. Every member will have them in varying degrees of sophistication. The developmental and learning process of individuals as well as of the team should be to focus on the continual attention to enhancing and improving the interactional processes of team members with the team as a whole.

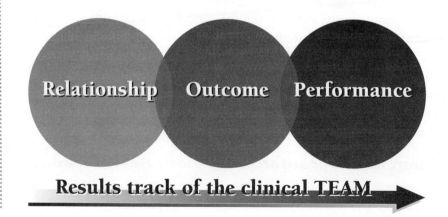

THREE ELEMENTS OF EVALUATION

Relationship   Outcome   Performance

Results track of the clinical TEAM

ELEMENTS OF EVALUATION

A further expectation is that the individual is able to work well with implementing the group's processes, the expectations of the group, and the clinical paths, critical pathways, care maps, and other processes that define the activities and expectations of the group. Certainly, team members must be able to commit to group decisions of which they were a part. Even though it may surely be recognized that certain individuals in a group may not necessarily always agree with the strategies, activities, and decisions of the group, because they are team members they inherently consent to implement the decisions of the group once those have been determined. They further agree to incorporate their energies and investment around the activities necessary to make the group process successful. This takes a level of maturity and insight that will be present at varying degrees of intensity in each member of the team.

The expectation is that each member has the basic skills and abilities to interact, problem solve, and achieve the goals of the team in an effective and meaningful way.

The ability to collaborate in an ongoing way and to delineate and do the work of the team is an important evaluative element in the individual's appraisal by the team. Team members should be able to remove barriers to the relationships they have with each other. Each team member should know that in the learning plan, the performance evaluation, and the improvement process, the clinical delivery system and all of the elements that enumerate it, there is evidence that the individual is able to embrace the issues that arise in implementing the activities of patient care and to directly and honestly confront them as a member of the team in a way that invests the team members in solution seeking, problem solving, and advancing practice. The attitude and expectation should be one of enthusiasm, engagement, and excitement. The ability of the individual to achieve positive solutions in a "win-win" environment is critical to the viability of the team-based approach and team-based activities.

TEAM EFFECTIVENESS CYCLE

OUTCOME
Clinical process
Protocols
Competence
Performance

RELATIONSHIPS
Member relations
Process skills
Group dynamics
Role clarity

PERFORMANCE
Expectations
Measures
Evaluation
Discipline

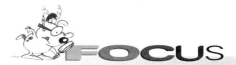

FOCUS

Collaboration requires that team members be proficient at managing their relationships with each other. Such management demands a level of maturity that includes the ability to:
- *Work through personal differences*
- *Problem solve using critical processes*
- *Use continuous quality methods*
- *Make personal changes when indicated*
- *Facilitate others' and own growth activities*

The relationship format for all teams is "win-win." If competition between players for control, ego, rewards, benefit, or position operates at the expense of the team congruence, outcomes suffer and the team ethic dissipates. When that is gone—so is the team.

TEAM COMMUNICATION PROCESS

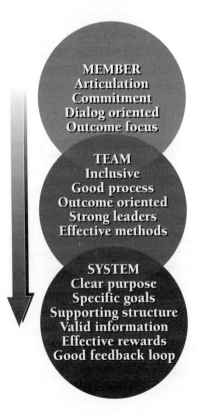

MEMBER
Articulation
Commitment
Dialog oriented
Outcome focus

TEAM
Inclusive
Good process
Outcome oriented
Strong leaders
Effective methods

SYSTEM
Clear purpose
Specific goals
Supporting structure
Valid information
Effective rewards
Good feedback loop

In team-based systems the ability to communicate effectively is critical to the success of the team. Communication is the life blood of the team. It is central to the ongoing effectiveness of team relationships. If an individual is not able to articulate, integrate, and communicate effectively in the team, the team begins to break down in fundamental ways and its outcomes and expectations remain unfulfilled. Therefore all members should be able to communicate and articulate their role, expectations, communication, and responses in a meaningful way. Expression of their thoughts and feelings, notions, and creativities should be communicated in an effective and constructive manner. Nonconfrontation, ability to facilitate integration, and ability to engage team members in a viable and meaningful way are essential constituents of effective communications.

The individual should also be able to use the information infrastructure and communications system effectively. In team-based approaches it is no longer a legitimate excuse for team members to say, "I didn't know." The obligation for knowing rests with the individual. The obligation of the communication infrastructure is to make sure that knowing is possible. Therefore measurement of the individual's ability to receive and to convey information, to express the self clearly and well, to articulate feelings, thoughts, and notions, and to act consistently as a contributing member of the team in its deliberations will be critical evaluative criteria for the individual team member's contribution.

Consistent with communication measurement and interpersonal skills, and identification with the team's expectation and outcomes, is the requisite that members be able to relate specifically to the subscriber, patient, or service receiver in an effective and meaningful way. Some practitioners have a history of not being able to communicate well with those they serve. This is untenable in a team-based approach. Those who are served have a right to expect that the interaction, intersection, communication, and relationship with the service provider will be positive, meaningful, and considerate. All relationship to service receivers and those who are a part of their network is a critical part of the effectiveness and efficacy of the team-based approach. The point-of-service demands that those who are served are at the center of the organizational system, and as members of the system continuously hopeful of improvements in the quality of life or in their health process. Each person has the right to expect that the provider will be concerned, interested, and sensitive to all of his or her health care needs. Therefore the individual is involved in advancing the relationship with the patient or consumer, the education of the consumer, and developing and refining the relational and interactional processes between consumers and providers within the health care delivery system.

ACCOUNTABILITY AND PERFORMANCE

Accountability is the cornerstone of performance. While teams have accountability to achieve the outcomes to which they are directed, team members have specific accountabilities whose exercise operates in fulfillment of the purposes, mission, and outcomes of the team and the organizational system. Therefore each team member has specific accountabilities that numerate his or her role and contribution to the work of the team and of the system. These accountabilities should be outcome defined, clearly enumerated, well articulated, and part of the team's performance evaluation of the individual's contribution to the team's work. Accountability relates to the expectations for performance of the individual in terms of the outcomes to which that performance is directed. The outcomes must be clear and the accountability in outcome language must be specific and understandable to every member of the team. It can therefore serve as the criteria on which the team measures the appropriate behaviors and practices of the individual discipline.

Accountabilities arise out of the discipline that should also be a part of the evaluation. The discipline member is responsible to make it clear to other members of the team what those elements of the discipline are that should be part of the evaluation process to that the team members can be engaged. Using these accountabilities for performance evaluation provides an objective template and framework for other team

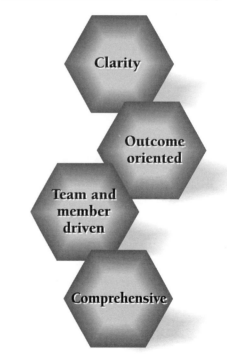

ACCOUNTABILITY ELEMENTS

Clarity

Outcome oriented

Team and member driven

Comprehensive

Accountability requires ownership on the part of every team member in relationship to each other.

Accountability is always expressed in terms of the outcomes that are achieved, not the processes that are implemented.

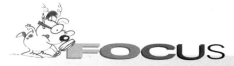

The team is now the basic unit of work. It creates a real challenge for leadership to see process and structure in the context of team-driven processes. To do so means the following:

- *No more individual performance evaluations out of the context of the team process*
- *More rewards directed toward the team rather than simply the individual*
- *Better generation of information toward the point-of-service (team)*
- *Leadership development in the skills of facilitation, coordination, integration, and mentoring*

members to look at the behavior of any one team member. It also serves as a mechanism for delineating the expectations for performance and for articulating corrective action wherever that is indicated in the performance evaluation process.

Each of the above elements serves as a discipline or framework that team members can use for evaluating the relationship of individual team members with the team. When integrated with the team's obligation for measuring its performance against the outcomes to which it is directed, it serves as a complete performance evaluation framework for team-based activities. The two levels of evaluation articulated at the beginning of this chapter-the individual's relationship to the team and the team's relationship to its outcomes-are therefore adequately addressed within the context of a whole systems approach to team-based evaluation processes.

The mechanisms of evaluation in team-based systems are new and therefore challenging. The dynamics of team-based performance evaluation and improvement, as well as individual relationships to team performance improvement activities, are clearly different from those experienced in the past by individuals in an organization. The movement from individual performance evaluation to team-based systems brings with it much adjustment, challenge, and noise in expectations, performance, and evaluation processes. The centerpiece of all evaluation is the accountability that drives the performance of individuals and the activities of the group.

Enumerating accountabilities in light of the clinical processes and the expectations of the team becomes the framework within which all performance gets defined and all performance evaluation and improvement unfold. Linking the concept of evaluation and improvement to the outcomes of the team and the organization's mission and purposes creates a systematic, cyclical approach to team activities and performance evaluation. Here again, systems process and dynamics drive the character of understanding performance evaluation. It becomes less critical to enumerate performance deficits of an individual and more important for identifying the developmental, interactional, and outcome-oriented requisites for ensuring effective delivery of care and sustainable outcomes. It is the systematic approach, a cyclical integrated dynamic in a team-based system, that creates an organizational structure and process that forms the framework supporting the point-of-service. Good team foundations ensure consistent achievement of clinical outcomes and a constant attention to the improvement of performance and the delivery of quality services.

Bibliography

Allred C et al: Case management: the relationship between structure and enment, *Nursing Economics* 13(1):32-42, 1995.

Allred C et al: A cost effective analysis of acute care case management outcomes, *Nursing Economics* 13(3):129-136, 1995.

Bowers M, Swan J, Koehler W: What attributes determine quality and satisfaction with health care delivery? *Health Care Management Review* 19(4):49-55, 1995.

Center HI: *The medical outcomes and guidelines sourcebook,* New York, Faulker and Grey, 1994.

Eckhart J: Costing out nursing service: examining the research, *Nursing Economics* 11(2):91-98, 1993.

Gustafson D, Helstad C, Hung CF: The total costs of illness: a metric for health care reform, *Hospital and Health Services Administration* 40(1):154-171, 1995.

Harris M: Clinical and financial outcomes in patient care in a home health agency, *Journal of Nursing Quality Assurance* 5(2):41-49, 1991.

Kaluzny A, McLaughlin C, Kibbe D: Quality improvement: beyond the institution, *Hospital and Health Services Administration* 40(1):172-187, 1995.

Kerr M, Rudy E, Daly B: Human response patterns to outcomes in the critically ill patient, *Journal of Nursing Quality Assurance* 5(2):32-40, 1991.

Kritek P: *Negotiating at an uneven table,* San Francisco, Berrett-Koehler, 1994.

Leavenworth G: Quality costs less, *Business and Health* 12(3):7-11, 1994.

Longo D: The impact of outcomes measurement on the hospital-physician relationship, *Topics in Health Care Financing* 20(4):63-74, 1994.

Niven D: When times get tough, what happens to TQM? *Harvard Business Review* 71(3):20-34, 1993.

Parker G: *Cross functional teams,* San Francisco, Jossey-Bass, 1994.

Porter-O'Grady T, Tornabeni J: Outcomes of shared governance: impact on the organization, *Seminars for Nurse Managers,* 1(2):63-73, 1993.

Program FN: *A study of the outcomes of nutritional programs on the cost of later Medicaid outlays,* Washington, DC, Department of Agriculture, 1990.

Rooks J et al: Outcomes of care in birth centers, *New England Journal of Medicine* 321:1804-1811, 1990.

Taguchi G: Quality imperatives, *Harvard Business Review* 70(1):65-71, 1990.

Western P: QA/QI and nursing competence: a combined model, *Nursing Management* 25(3):44-46, 1994.

Zander K: *Managing outcomes through collaborative care: care mapping and case management,* Chicago, American Hospital Publishing, 1995.

Index

319